*To Linda
with all my best wishes
Jenni.*

Trapped

Living with Gender Dysphoria

By Jennifer Brown

First published in 2007 by Jennifer Brown

*PO Box xxxxxxxxx
Bridgwater, Somerset*

© 2007 Jennifer Brown. All rights reserved.

The right of Jennifer to be identified as the author of this work has been asserted by her in accordance with the Copyright, Designs and Patents Act 1988.

All rights reserved. No part of this publication may be reproduced, stored in a retrieval system, or transmitted, in any form or by any means, without prior written permission of the publisher, nor be otherwise circulated in any form of binding or cover other than that which it is published and without a similar condition including this condition being imposed on the subsequent purchaser.

ISBN: 978-0-9557207-0-3

Cover design by RPM Print & Design

*Printed and bound in Great Britain by
RPM Print & Design
2-3 Spur Road, Quarry Lane, Chichester, West Sussex
PO19 8PR*

Foreword

This book could almost be called Version 1. It is my story, a story of my life living with a medical condition that for most of my adult life I did not know I had, something I had not heard of or knew existed and a condition my brain had fought to keep consigned to my subconscious by propelling me thorough life at a manic pace pursuing goals and objectives with almost obsessional focussed single-mindedness. It is an evolving story though, as my life adapts to living with or recovering from the worst psychological effects of this condition so there will be more to the story and as medical and neural researchers now on an almost weekly basis seems to unearth more and more of the complex biological interactions that cause this condition to appear then also the story will change and evolve.

This book actually started life as a food and wine guide to the pubs and restaurants in the area of London where my apartment is!! I was half way through this blockbuster, had a couple of potential publishers eagerly interested, was looking forward to retiring on the proceeds for the rest of my life as a 25 stone alcoholic having eaten and drunk my way up Chiswick High Road when disaster struck. I lost the manuscript. Then, by one of those awful heart-stopping moments of great melodrama, whilst copying the backup onto my laptop I corrupted both, back-up disk AND hard disk. Bemoaning my fate to a friend, someone who herself has written books on human turmoil, it was suggested that perhaps someone might be telling me something and I should instead write a book on Gender Dysphoria as I at least had a first-hand perspective.

Being a Christian I take note when it is suggested someone is "trying to tell me something" so there and then I set about writing a book on just what being Gender dysphoric means to people. I originally envisaged overlying my first-hand experiences with more general "Types of Gender Dysphoric person" but quickly realised there is no specific "Type". Firstly the whole population is too small. The Government estimates there are only 7,000 or so people like me in the whole of the population generally, males and females.

The next realisation to hit home was almost everyone I talked to, read about or discussed in general terms had different experiences. There is no "typical gender Dysphoric person", just some rather general reactions and. unfortunately, a large proportion of death by suicide. Some, like me, knew from childhood they were different, others, unlike me, were able to articulate why and "come out" in childhood. Some, like me, tried to commit suicide in childhood and we will never know accurately how many succeeded for they are not here to record their reasons why.

Some were able to repress feelings throughout most of their adult life, others realised early on. There is one common characteristic of those who repress well into middle age and that is the manic, almost self-destructive, "more macho than most, constant need to prove themselves over and over again" type of behaviour, as it certainly applied to me. Why, as I was to learn, there are so many who were either once, or still serving, in jobs such as the SAS, Military specialist operations units, police tactical units (SWAT in the USA), Whilst writing this book an officer in the parachute regiment, decorated for bravery, declared he was transitioning, and also in the same period an ex-military special operations person who was bodyguard to the rich and famous before deciding to swap flak jacket for something a bit more feminine announced her transition. Others are successful in other fields such as sport, in business, the arts or technology, a restless driven anxiety driving them on into a constant "proving oneself" workaholic fervour. Again, given that many of us follow dangerous careers or pastimes, go through life at a pace guaranteed to cause a breakdown of some description or other, or are driven into a state of anguish that often becomes suicidal, just how many premature deaths occur due to an undercurrent of gender Dysphoria can only remain as conjecture.

For many the core of what has been wrong with them for most of their life is only discovered after some form of catastrophic breakdown, or in my case the final breakdown after many. Some its more overt, a lifetime of transvestism type activity metamorphoses into a realisation that rather than being a man enjoying occasionally his female side, they are in fact a female allowing their natural femininity to be released when possible and being female is the natural gender role, although perhaps surprisingly to the outside observer very few gender Dysphoric people who undergo transition do so after arriving at the conclusion they are living in the wrong gender as a progression from transvestism. With most it is a realisation that continues from childhood or arrives "out of nowhere" in adulthood with no previous transvestic or cross-dressing background.

With no "typical template" to work off I then decided I should use my life, my experiences as an illustration of what it is to live with Gender Dysphoria. It is my story but written to give hope to others, not just people suffering with the same condition but to anyone who through no fault of their own find themselves belonging to a minority that is little understood, seen to be different and often having to confront prejudice and bigotry, It could actually reflect many peoples lives. a life with a difficult beginning, a dark and terrible middle but a happy ending, in fact a life ultimately of happiness with the realisation of the joy of happiness being forged and tempered through the fires of dark and difficult times.

It is written as an autobiographical account but it is not a biography as such. Events and behaviour patterns not particularly related to the actions of someone struggling with a deep internal unhappiness and anguish are not discussed or elaborated on, this is an observation of those thoughts and feelings, and associated behaviour patterns, that affected one particular individual as they struggled to come to terms with all the stresses of being "different" even when the brain would not allow that difference to manifest itself or become consciously apparent. Where possible I have attempted to protect those who may wish anonymity or employers who may not wish to be disclosed therefore details of my life as it relates to individuals and employers are at best kept vague and if not relevant to illustrating the main theme of this book are omitted altogether. Also some incidents that could identify others or identify circumstances that could affect currently ongoing issues have either been modified, omitted or had dates changed.

When I look at the happiness I have now in my life and the various chapters that have led me here I realise just how fortunate I am. I an surrounded by friends and family who have given me unconditional love and support, a partner who for over half my life has been everything anyone could want in their lives, I live in a stable safe country where we take freedom of speech and freedom to worship for granted, I have never experienced the personal disruption of a war at home, I have access to some of the finest medical treatment on the planet. It would be very easy for me to complain that "society does not accept me" when in fact I live in one of the most tolerant and peaceful societies on the planet.

My good fortune can be compared starkly with those peoples across the planet who face only genocidal hatred, who for no reason of their own face murder, mutilation and starvation just because they are the wrong colour, worship in a different way or come from the wrong tribe. Today some of the most desperately oppressed people are facing the evil of genocide in what is probably the worst humanitarian disaster on the planet occurring now, at this minute, in the Darfur region of Western Sudan. I am therefore pledging £2.00, effectively my margin after publication costs, for every copy of this book sold to Christian aid agencies helping those desperately unfortunate peoples.

Table of Contents

Chapter 1: Into the prison Born 1
Chapter 2: Childhood: Development 5
Chapter 3: Childhood: Crisis 13
Chapter 4: Proving himself 23
Chapter 5: The business career 37
Chapter 6: Recovery 49
Chapter 7: Back to business 59
Chapter 8: Charity begins, and ends, at home 65
Chapter 9: Emergence 79
Chapter 10: No longer David, not quite Jenni 91
Chapter 11: Transition 99
Chapter 12: Now 115
Chapter 13: Jo's story 123
Chapter 14: Faith 133
Chapter 15: From the outside looking in 143
Chapter 16: Reflections 153
Acknowledgments 167

Dedication

I was stuck when it came to dedicating this book. Who should it be dedicated to?

Obviously it should be dedicated to my Jo, my partner, my wife, my soul mate, my best friend, the person who has stood beside me for 37 years and who has been through hell and back to keep standing by me. But there were so many others, just how could I mention them all, how could I even start to draw up a list?

Then it came to me. A few weeks before this book was finished it was my 60th birthday, a big party had been planned to be held in a restaurant with a capacity for 60 guests but this was causing a problem. There were in fact 120 people on the guest list, people who I know I could say were friends in every sense of the word, people who have lived with me through some of the darkest times in my life, people who have had to accept the bizarre changes in my life but people who have been called upon to be counted and have not been found wanting.

In the end I reasoned that with my party being held on a bank holiday weekend and at the start of a long school holiday most people would be away anyway so it was safe to invite all 120. 80 actually turned up but we all squeezed in and the party went wonderfully well.

This book is dedicated though to all those 120 people on the list. Jo, my family and Jo's family in their entirety, friends of long standing, neighbours and friends from the small village community where we live, my church family from the congregation of the small parish church where we worship, people from business where business relationships have blossomed into firm friendships, health professionals, medical, dental and therapists from other disciplines whose professional care has matured into friendship, those friends who have only ever met the Jennifer Brown version but know of the past version and his history, to all those 120 people, from the bottom of my heart thank you, thank you whoever you are, from wherever you have come from, thank you for giving me the privilege of being able to call you my friend.

Chapter 1:
Into the prison Born

David was born on the 8th of May 1947. Two years earlier to the day the nation had rejoiced as it was officially proclaimed that war with Germany was over. There was Victory in Europe and forever more the 8th May was to be remembered as VE day.

These were not easy times for the nation generally and for David's parents they had been especially difficult. At the time of conception they already had another daughter, Shirley, less than two years old and were living in cramped accommodation with David's paternal grandparents.

A few weeks into foetal development and David's grandparents decided that a pregnant woman with a young child was too much for the cramped accommodation and asked his Mother, also Shirley, to find somewhere else to live. For weeks she tramped the streets pushing the young Shirley in a pushchair and with the fatigue and sickness associated with a child growing inside her until finally they found somewhere, it was one of those ubiquitous dwellings called a "prefab", short for prefabricated house, that seemed to sprout up on every available bit of cleared land in war torn London, and this prefab was one of two side by side on a plot of land hastily cleared of piles of rubble that had been previously been deposited there by a German landmine destroying a large Victorian house that had once stood proudly on that plot of land.

Today attention would have been paid to the pollution risks. The land was soaked with nitrates from the explosives the bombs were packed with, broken sewers had leaked their filthy contents into the ground and the detritus of bombed building rubble was all around but in the desperate conditions caused by 5 years of war and intensive bombing these were issues that did not matter then. Inside the deeply stressed mother, living in heavily polluted surroundings, certain parts of the foetal brain of the developing child entered their most critical development stage.

David was born at home, a relatively straightforward birth other than he was a rather large baby weighing in at over 10 pounds and the Doctor, having had a quick glance at the genitalia, pronounced to the happy couple that they had a boy.

There was no discussion on the name. As David's mother had named his sister after herself so David's father felt it his manly right to assert himself and rushed off down to the registry office to register the male infant with his own name.

Being seen to be "Manly" was very important to David's father. This was at the height of gender polarisation in British society, where men were men and women were women and no blurring of the edges. These were days of hard manual labour, of heavy industries such as steelmaking, shipbuilding, coalmining, rail and road car manufacturing etc..

Two bloody hard fought world wars had heightened gender polarisation with "men going off to fight" but by the end of the Second World War the cracks were beginning to show. Towards the end of the first world war women drafted into previously men dominated industries started to wear trousers and by the 1920's the wearing of trousers by women was taking hold despite stiff opposition from a male-dominated society. The Suffragettes had achieved emancipation and women now had the right to vote. The drain in manpower of the second world war caused yet more women to take their place in previously men only jobs and each of the armed forces had its own female wing, the WAAFS, WRNS and WRACs and women were contributing to the final sacrifice given in wartime by so many, the toll of heavy bombing raids on dockyards, airfields and military bases exacting a heavy price.

David's father was part of one of a succession of post war generations that would resist this growing emancipation. Men had to be Men, boys had to be boys and his son was going to be encouraged in every possible way to be a boy's boy growing up to be a Man's man.

There was one problem with all of this. David was in fact Female, a Female trapped in the prison of a male body with nurturing and social acceptance becoming the jailors.

Chapter 2
Childhood: Development

David was born when what we call Gender, our identity, what we are, how we understand ourselves and how we relate to each other in society, was considered to be a product of nurture. We were either physically born Male or Female and depending on those physical characteristics our brains "learnt" to identify as male or female and our behaviour and relationships with each other duly followed.

It is now known that Gender and Physical sexual characteristics are two separate components of our whole and that our gender is largely developed by the time we are born. Various processes during the period of foetal development act upon the developing brain so at birth it is largely programmed to know which physical body it is in, either a male or a female. Brains of typical males and typical females are also physically different and post-mortems carried out on people like David has revealed that their brains have the typical structure normally found in people of the opposite physical sex, in David's case a physically female brain in a physically male body and a brain that is innately psychologically female as well.

To most of us this is a confusing issue that we have no need to concern ourselves with for our brains and physical bodies are in harmony, all those processes during foetal development ensuring that the brain of the new-born infant is entirely congruent with the physical characteristics. We do not even have to think about two processes being in joint harmony, same as we do not have to think about the miracle of our hearts and lungs being in such perfect harmony that 20 times a minute we can breathe without difficulty. Should that process falter, even for a fraction of a second those separate process of heart and lung were not synchronised, then our lives would be rendered a misery of breathing difficulties, heart strain and other discomforts.

So it is for people like David, the lack of harmony between brain and body causing a deep unhappiness that gives rise to the medical condition called gender dysphoria. David was born gender dysphoric. No one can say why. The most accepted theory is that it was due to a hormonal accident at about 16 weeks of development that caused hormonal signals to be crossed. It is known that this is the time the brain starts to develop as male or female, it is at this time that hormonal bursts from the developing foetus increase dramatically and something goes wrong at this time. There are a variety of theories of what can go wrong including combinations of amongst other things maternal stress and nitrate pollutants but whatever the cause, whatever happened, it was an accident and fortunately an accident that only occurs in about 1 in 8,000 of the population.

David's brain does not want to be reminded of a childhood where he had no control, was forced to behave and form associations that were contrary to how he thought and felt and how possibly he deeply ached to be something different so childhood memories are very sparse and episodic.. This, some therapists, call "lost childhood syndrome" so specific instances throughout his childhood have to remain as unrecalled episodes.

Those memories that can be recalled and whatever observations and conclusions that are made here can be documented, supported by known facts and dates, to ensure there is no selective memory recall or no post-childhood misinterpretation. With what was to happen to David late in his adult life he was more anxious than anyone that any conclusions drawn must be correct and right as for the rest of his life, or at least his happiness for the rest of his life, was to depend on getting it right.

By the age of 9 examples of behaviour that can be remembered point to a child that often sought solitary comfort, wanting to be on his own, prone to going for long solitary walks or in his bedroom holding animated conversations with his teddy or an imaginary friend. He enjoyed cooking and messing about in the kitchen and baking cakes became almost on obsession. All these activities were frowned upon by a father who was expecting his son to be a "Boys boy". He felt himself to be under almost unremitting pressure to go and mix with the boys on the street corner, something that was totally foreign to his nature, to the way he wanted to be. It was not that he was ill equipped to be a boy, he was highly competitive and good at football and other team games although poor eyesight often hindered his ability to coordinate hand and eye, he had a hair trigger temper, was naturally aggressive and was good in a fight, although of diminutive height he was quite stocky. All these attributes however did not matter, quite simply doing "typical boy things", even things he was good at, was just totally foreign to his nature.

He was an emotional child. Tears of compassion would easily flow; animals or people being hurt would rapidly bring tears to his eyes but in a boy attributes of emotional compassion are not qualities to be welcomed and this was just another source of approbation and increased the feelings of being different.

At this time there were other indications of a deep seated unhappiness and psychological disturbance. Like many infants he sucked his thumb but this habit intensified rather than decreased as he grew older, drawing sometimes sneering and bullying remarks from his father and often being teased by other boys.

He recalls on many occasions waking up with headache and being very afraid to open his eyes, probably attacks of the acute migraine that he would be diagnosed as suffering with 11 years later and would blight him throughout his adult life.

He can recall having dreams at this stage that were quite disturbing. He would dream of being in a family scene, e.g. a birthday party, but isolated, everyone being formed into other groups, but not him, always on the edge, never being noticed, never being included. His sense of isolation was growing, for the first time these dreams was expressing thoughts he had hitherto been unable to rationalise, that he was different, that he was socially dislocated from his peer group, that he didn't belong anywhere. He does not recall at any time of wanting to be a girl, just of not wanting to be a boy, of knowing he wasn't a boy.

Another recollection he has is of a place of solitary retreat. Near their home was a small park, Myatts fields, fringed by ornamental bushes and evergreens with various benches dotted around it there was one favourite place. This was a half moon inset, cut into the widest part of the evergreen and shrub border, and in this inset arranged around this semi-circle were four benches. Behind these benches were a laurel bushes and rhododendrons and a willow tree with branches touching to the ground. The inside of this natural hollow was a perfect hiding place, concealed from view and protected by those benches from anyone walking close by. This became his den, a place he could retreat to, unnoticed, and just be with himself, talking to his imaginary friend, to

Trapped

God, to anyone whom he thought would understand him in a world where he felt so misunderstood and so isolated.

Nearly half a century later, as a wounded animal retreats to its lair, so as an adult again struggling with those same feelings of social dislocation and isolation, he would again be drawn to this bolthole of solitary isolation.

David's parents could not be faulted. Dad could, and often did, resort to sneering taunts, especially when his son displayed any sort of behaviour that could in any sense be called "sissy" but this was a product of the times and an intensely gender-polarised society. Any other child not having those deep feelings of being different would just have gone with it, accepted it and let it pass but for David struggling with such internal conflict these taunts could be deeply wounding and just increased his sense of isolation. In a way also it deepened what was already a keen sense of self-reliance, to depend on no one but himself for support in times of struggle, something that was to become a major strength of his when it came to surviving his adult years.

Mum had to work part time, in fact Mum worked as hard as any Mum could, that was the economic reality of the times, so David rarely had an opportunity to release those inner fears.

At the age of 10 this deep unhappiness was triggered into starting an out of control downward tumble into an emotional black hole and would result in him being mentally scarred for the rest of his life. He went on a holiday with the school to the Isle of Wight.

Up to this point his discomfort with acting the role of a boy and doing it well enough to earn parental and social pride and pleasure had been tempered by being allowed to find solitary comfort, to escape from the pressures of the crowd by indulging in those activities where he could just lose himself in his thoughts, thoughts that expressed openly would of earned severe parental and institutional displeasure. Now there was no escape. For ten days he would be forced to sleep in a large, crowded all-boy dormitory, forced to eat breakfast from a large, crowded all-boy dining room, spend the day indulging in rowdy boy only activities. Desperately afraid to be seen as different he would overcompensate by being the rowdiest, the noisiest, and the most aggressive and yet this would backfire for it would earn disapproval and admonishment from the teachers in charge. The no win situation intensified profoundly his feelings of being different, being dislocated, being abnormal, of being unwanted.

For the rest of his life the scars from this episode would persist, persist so much that even many years later as a respected and successful businessman being invited to exotic places to participate in a three day corporate stag weekends or "jolly's away" packed full of typical male things to do would so prey on his mind that sleep and an ability to concentrate would suffer, just as it would do in this stage of his life. So serious would the fears of having to go away for "blokes weekends or corporate events" that his efforts to fined excuses not to go would even veer towards self-harm or, at the extreme, self-destruction to avoid such an event.

Soon after the trip to the Isle of Wight the 11 plus and change of schools beckoned. He was considered a bright child, outstandingly good at mental arithmetic, reading and writing and writing had become one of his greatest passions, especially the dream-like nonsense of childhood prose, although again writing silly stories was not an activity welcomed by a Father wanting a boys-boy to grow into a mans-man so writing was almost a covert and secret activity. Passing the 11 plus and gaining a seat at grammar school should have been a foregone conclusion.

It wasn't.

By now the deepening sense of being different and not being able to conform had, after that dreaded school holiday, accelerated into feelings of a complete lack of self-worth and a complete lack of self belief. The dreams of isolation and social dislocation had now had introduced into them a further disturbing element, they now sometimes ended up with David being accepted into a group, being happy, only in these endings he was dressed as a girl, was with other girls and had a girls name, always the same name, Jennifer. Where this name came from is a mystery, no family member or friend had this name, but in those dreams it was always the name Jennifer he had whenever he was happy.

For someone so wanting to fulfil parental, social and academic aspirations this was the worst possible thing. No matter what David may have felt inside, or deep down in his mind knew himself to be, any thought, feeling or action of femininity would be a disgrace and bring on sneering approbation. The fear of showing any form of femininity now intensified, with it the disturbance in his mind intensified, concentration suffered, he failed his 11 plus.

Chapter 3
Childhood: Crisis

That Autumn, aged 11, he started at a new school, a central school, not good enough for a Grammar school but still considered to have an O-level brain he was sent to what was an in-between school, this being before comprehensive schools had become the norm.

At this school his misery deepened. Being there rather than at a Grammar school like his Sister deepened his sense of worthlessness and of being a failure. The school prided itself on its excellence at sport and someone good at football and rugby was naturally expected to give up evenings and weekends to participate in games and as he was encouraged to do so then his ability to escape into solitary isolation diminished. His concentration at school suffered as the dreams persisted and his sense of isolation and social dislocation deepened, the fear of showing femininity in any way possible caused him to become aggressive and withdrawn.

He was also considered to be "lazy", or a "failure" for other reasons. He was someone outstandingly good at mental arithmetic, someone who on more than one occasion was top of his school, at the age of 11 proving himself better than the brightest 16 year olds, so it was naturally assumed he was equally good at other types of maths and by extension should be good at physics. He wasn't. In fact he was then, and is now, a complete dismal failure. This failure at extended logic subjects such as geometry, calculus, physics etc. was considered to be due to a lack of application. "Could do better" was repeatedly written on his report to be taken home, taken home to a Father who, wanting his son to be a boys boy, a winner at everything, displayed his dissatisfaction with bouts of violent temper aimed towards his son.

It was only in later years was he able to explain this anomaly, explaining how with mental arithmetic he could visualise numbers as patterns, patterns that when matched with other patterns merged to form the answer. He did not solve arithmetical puzzles solely depending on the logical centres of his brain, he solved them depending a lot on the visual-spatial centres. Logic centres are often seen as more strongly developed in atypical males, visual and spatial centres as something normally more strongly developed in atypical females.

Finally, berated at home for not doing all those "Boy" things he should be doing, berated at school for poor performance, desperately fighting feelings of isolation, failure and confusion as to what he was he ran away from home.

He did this three times. The first time was an unplanned affair, a few hours retreat to his place of sanctuary in Myatts fields, but it was a cold, wet, windy November night and it was not long before he was trudging forlornly home. The second time he was picked up by the police whilst trudging aimlessly alone, lost in his thoughts and pain, along the streets and roads of London a few miles from his home.

The third time was a better planned and determined attempt to escape from his personal hell forever, no less a meticulous plan for stowing away on one of the great ocean liners to America where he had some loose form of plan in his head of trying to find a job as a street kid, working on the markets of New York City he had read about, doing odd jobs, until old enough to pass as an adult and eventually apply for immigration as an established alien. He had read it all in books, whether the accounts were true of false he had convinced himself his plan would succeed and he set about planning its execution.

First he had to "escape" from home for more than just a few hours. He knew of a day nursery near by, flimsy windows that could be opened easily, a place of refuge for a couple of nights to take him to the right day for when one of the great ocean liners was about to leave harbour. He then had to get to that harbour and board the ship. His plan was simple. The day prior to departure a boat train service left Waterloo station bound for the ocean terminal at Southampton. The night before he planned to arrive at Waterloo station, climb the fence running alongside the platform at the quietest time of night, conceal himself on the platform until the train pulled in from the sidings, then board the empty train concealing himself until it was full of passengers and ready to depart. Once at Southampton he had a loose plan in his head, formulated from various books he had read about the cargo carried on board these huge ships, to hide within a pallet of cargo and board the ship. From then on it was going to be an exercise of "living off his wits" until safely ashore in New York,

It all went well at first, he escaped from home climbing out of a bedroom window when his parents thought he was asleep gaining a precious few hours before his disappearance was detected. The entry into the nursery proved to be easy, he was away at daybreak before arrival of any staff, his nocturnal occupancy went unnoticed, and he spent that day travelling on the London underground until late at night. He then returned to the nursery for another overnight stay, repeated his travels on the London underground before making his way to Waterloo Station.

As midnight approached he was able to scale the fence unnoticed, find himself on the boat train platform and squirming underneath a platform bench was able to spend the night concealed until the train pulled in from the sidings.

However his attempt to smuggle himself onto an ocean liner and escape to the USA was finally foiled when a station cleaning attendant discovered him huddled underneath the bench only hours before the opportunity to get on the train going to the ocean terminus at Southampton arose. He was taken into police custody, identified as the child a "missing, at risk" bulletin had been issued for and returned by police car to await collection in the early hours of the morning by a tired and gaunt father. Even though his relationship with his Dad was often stormy and he often suffered from his father's sneering and verbally abusive tongue, the memory of the strain and tiredness on his Dad's face and the feelings of guilt this brought on him would remain a painful memory for the rest of his life.

He was hauled before the juvenile courts and even in that harsh environment of the day it was realised that here was a child that was profoundly psychologically disturbed. Rather than the custodial sentence to a place of punishment that was originally considered he was instead taken to a children's' home for observation, a two month period of residency

This confinement would have been disastrous but for a stroke of good fortune. The home largely acted as a foster home to children from broken backgrounds. These children used the home like any other home, going to a normal school during the day. The only residential school facilities that were provided were for educationally challenged children

Trapped

and soon the residential school faced a quandary. Here was someone of above average intelligence, sent there for confinement so could not be released for external schooling but far too advanced intellectually for the residential school to accommodate.

The compromise was self-education. For David this was heaven. All of the day, for every weekday, he was on his own, left to use the library for reading and learning purposes, encouraged by psychologists to write whatever he cared to write, no interaction with anyone else. For 8 hours a day five days a week he could dream away, be whoever he wanted to be and indulge his love of creative writing without any approbation from home.

He also had another stroke of good fortune at this home. At school David had befriended a shy, withdrawn boy of mixed race. This boy suffered in many ways. He had learning difficulties that led to him having a difficult time with teachers, his timidity would lead to him being bullied by other boys and his racial background, in an era when colour prejudice was rife and to be mixed race was the worst of all worlds made him a target for widespread abuse. Perhaps David recognised someone else who because he was "different" was struggling in society, or perhaps it was just his natural compassion for anyone less fortunate than those around. Either way he helped this boy with his schoolwork, helped defend him against the worst of the bullying and often spent hours listening as this child opened his heart to probably the only friend he had.

Now at this home it was David that needed a friend for he himself, separated for the day from the other boys, was seen as being "different" and was at the beginning to come in for some fearsome bullying. It did not last long. Of all the young residents in the home one stood out, a tall muscular mixed race teenager who was there with his younger brother, one of the oldest residents having just left school and now working and undoubtedly the biggest, toughest kid on the block. One day he intervened in a Dining hall fracas that was resulting in David getting pushed around. David was to find out that this boy was the older brother of David's friend and had heard all about him and what he had done for his brother. Roughly sorting out one or two of the other molester's he made it very well known then, and on other occasions, that David was his friend and anyone picking on David would be picking on him. There was to be no more trouble after that.

Twice he had to return back to the Juvenile court and twice the psychiatrists reported on a considerable improvement to the psychological and behavioural problems that had led him there in the first place and commented favourably on how his writings were allowing them to see into his mind and understand the causes of his unhappiness. Clearly they felt their therapy was successful but sadly they were wrong. In that age gender dysphoria was considered to be a mental aberration of a sexually mature adult and not considered as something that could occur in a sexually undeveloped child. Their examinations of David precluded looking for any form of gender unhappiness and David, desperately trying to conceal to himself and the outside world any fears he may have had about his gender identity was steering well clear of anything that may allude to those types of problems.

Eventually the court had to decide what to do. He couldn't be left in limbo forever on a permanent observation order. It was either secure confinement in less hospitable surroundings or return back home. This galvanised David into expressing how much better he felt, how he really wanted to go back to school, knuckle down and work hard, how he was missing home etc. The court relented and sent him home but for three years he was to be under the close supervision of the child psychology unit of a leading London clinic.

Trapped

Nothing had really changed. It was back to the misery, the unhappiness but then good news, the school he so hated was to be merged with another school in the area and together they were to move into a bright new purpose built multi-storey block. Then there was other good news. With the children getting older, and his sister coming into puberty, his parents decided it was time to move, a brand new home on a brand new tower block estate and instead of two bedrooms there was going to be three and he would have his own room, his own space. As he passed his 13th birthday there was at last light to lift the gloom.

That summer came and went and moving into a new home, new streets to explore, new bus routes to travel on and new parks to find solitude in all added to a major distraction to the nagging unhappiness. That summer his explorations had taken him to East Grinstead, exploring a footpath he came across a couple of rock climbers practicing their skills on a low rock outcrop, and after returning a few times more he finally plucked up the courage to ask for a go himself. The climbers were helpful, not only allowing him to use their equipment but also explaining how it all worked, what ropes to use, what knots to tie them with and other places locally he could go to. For the first time in his life he had met people he could relate to, he felt accepted and he felt at last that he was able to prove his masculinity.

During this Summer he found himself increasingly turning to someone that had always been there in his life. He had no particular Christian faith, just a sincere unshakeable view that God existed and the God he knew was a loving, wiser older friend, not the austere God of retribution so often portrayed in those days, especially by a clergy who at times appeared to be not that far removed from the inquisition. More and more he found that God was the only person he could talk to, the only person he could trust and more and more it was a simple childlike faith that kept him from believing he was in an unending hell. Not for the last time was he to find salvation in a simple faith.

Back at school that autumn and it was still hell but a lesser hell. Many of the teachers he found himself working with had come from the other school, one where many children were brought up in overcrowded, broken or abusive homes and where many children also had learning difficulties. These teachers specialised in helping children simply survive, educational achievement was secondary. Now for the first time he could develop a rapport with some of the teaching staff and could be motivated. His psychological history travelled with him and some teachers aware of his difficulties looked for different ways to find him the space they wisely detected he needed. Physical education was still mandatory, his relationship with the head of the P.E. Department was a difficult one but instead of being forced to partake in activities he clearly rebelled against he was allowed to choose other activities. For a few hours a week the school swimming pool provided for both his physical exercise and his bolt hole of isolation. There were still behavioural difficulties, still educational application difficulties but he was, with the help of some inspirational and dedicated teachers, surviving.

When he was 14 he was asked to be a house prefect. He was given a job to do, prepare the school hall for assembly in the morning. He seized this responsibility with relish, instead of dragging his feet to school and being permanently late he was now arriving an hour early. Instead of being forced to mingle with the other children in the playground he now had good cause to be inside on his own. The house he belonged to, one of four at the school, for the rest of the time he was there never once started assembly late, unlike the other three that rarely started on time. What was to become a feature of his adult life, an ability to distract him totally from the pain of everyday existence by becoming completely immersed in one project or another, was first manifested with his job as house prefect.

There was something else about becoming a house prefect. The house Master who had asked him was one of those inspirational teachers who had helped him survive on that return to school. This house Master also shared his faith, by asking David to prepare the house for assembly he was amongst all else showing faith not only in David but also sharing their common spiritual faith. It was a bond that David was never to forget and was often grateful to be reminded of.

Now something else was coming along to disturb him. He was beginning to enter puberty. His sexual orientation was to be solely attracted to girls, yet not feeling a "proper" boy he was becoming confused about sexual attraction and was becoming overwhelmed with feelings of inadequacy. One weekend in November, at the age of 15, events conspired to bring all the doubts he had ever harboured together. He does not recall the whole of the links in the chain of events but does recall again with being overwhelmed with feelings of social dislocation and being different, not belonging to any social group. It was on a Monday, he can recall that with accuracy for his mother would leave money on the sideboard before she went to work so he could pay for his school meals for the forthcoming week. However on this Monday he did not go to school, instead he went to the local chemists and bought two large bottles of aspirin with his school dinner money, went home and over the next two hours swallowed all the pills plus whatever was in the household medicine cabinet, over 100 of them. He then went for a walk to await unconsciousness and final relief from his pain. It never happened. Instead he was violently sick, started shivering and sweating, experienced dizzy spells and a buzzing in the ears and went home and told his mum.

The parental discussion as he lay in bed was to say nothing. His record of psychological disturbance was bad enough;

this would only make it worse. Over the next few weeks a couple of teachers at school were taken into confidence, one in particular took special care of David, making sure at every possible opportunity he could bring words of encouragement and motivation to him. Eventually the crisis in his mind eased, the end of his schooldays beckoned and the time when he could at long last take charge over his life was in sight. Childhood survival was over. He was now an active rock climber. had taken to responsibility with a work ethic that was unrivalled amongst his peer group, was obsessively driven to succeed beyond all expectations. He had begun to find the tools to allow him to bury any thoughts of being different, bury any questions as to why he felt that way, the tools to survive adulthood.

Chapter 4:
Proving himself

For most of David's peer group, the priority on leaving school was to find a job promising a career, go on to further education or follow mum or dad into a family trade such as the print or motor trade. David had no real idea what he had to do and following a career was secondary, finding an identity, a role in life, a path to follow was more important.

For the next few years he was to follow a career path that promised little in terms of financial reward, much in terms of leading to a broken and wrecked body and a path that was most definitely macho in terms of the high level physical danger he was to regularly face. In the course of various jobs he was to find himself at times languishing in "bored out of his skull" inactivity at home, travelling the world in frenzied activity at other times, sometimes arriving back at the home port of entry only to have a message giving him 10 minutes notice he was going out again, just as at school the bad boy who was to be given leadership responsibility at a very early age, knowing the loss of close and loved friends and finally have to re-evaluate his life starting almost from scratch again.

Almost with everything he touched, every posting he accepted he found himself being propelled up the ranks but he needed something else other than just career success. He had to prove to himself and to the world in general, beyond all reasonable doubt, that he was male, macho and masculine regardless of physical pain and mental exhaustion. Whilst most of his peer group were now progressing regular civilian careers, entering into apprenticeships, going on to further education David's view of regular work developed into seeing it as something that was only temporary, only a necessary inconvenience interrupting his drive to prove his masculinity, expressed through his climbing and mountaineering exploits, and only there for as long as necessary to provide for his many trips away from home and away from the fear of being seen to be different.. Whatever else his various career pathways were to offer in terms of physical and mental demands David had to make sure that for every single minute of free time and time between postings he was proving himself over and over again.

In those periods totally responsible for his own life he could climb whenever and wherever he chose to do. The Lake District of England became his second home, his little orange one-man mountain tent a familiar site in the rugged mountainous terrain, all his possessions packed into one large grey Bergen.

He attacked the hardest rock climbing routes with a passion but when not climbing he was never still, always looking for new challenges, new rock climbing routes, new places to trek to. Many of the climbs he attempted, what would have been a new routes, first ascents that at the time were considered to be at the leading edge of technical ability, were to many others considered to be over the edge of acceptable limits of safety and either never got started or were quickly abandoned. His climbing had an abandon in it, a disregard for his own safety that exceeded the norm and that manic ferocious driven energy that had first become apparent in his school prefect days drove him on to ever extreme exploits. As at school he was popular, a regular member of a mountain rescue team and a first choice partner for many to climb with but still he yearned for solitude. As if returning home night after night to the isolation of his one-man tent was not enough he would periodically pack all his possessions into his enormous rucksack and disappear into the wilderness, not being seen for days, sometimes weeks.

Sometimes this trekking would have unforeseen results. One day he was returning back to his usual campsite, his heavily loaded rucksack draining energy, night rapidly falling. He decided to stop a couple of miles short of his destination for the night. He found a sheepfold, an open sided square consisting of low dry-stone walling erected to give sheep somewhere to shelter from the harsh winter winds. He unfolded his groundsheet and sleeping bag and curled up in this sheepfold and was soon asleep.

The following morning he awoke to bright sunshine but as he unwrapped himself from the warm snugness of his sleeping bag he noticed something terrible had happened overnight. All his exposed skin had turned black. As he stared in horror at his black skin he noticed it move. Sheep not only use sheepfolds for shelter, they also use them as handy places to scratch themselves and get rid of the irritating tics that cause their skin to itch. This sheepfold was alive with tics who had found a nice warm habitat to transfer themselves on to. In desperation he peeled off his clothes. Nearby was a mountain stream and oblivious to the cold early morning ambient temperature and the icy water of the stream with not a stitch of clothing on he plunged into it to rid himself of his unwanted guests. The cold took his breath away but it was going to be just one of those days.

From around a bend in the footpath he could hear singing. The location he had chosen for his impromptu overnight accommodation was a few hundred yards from an outdoor pursuits centre used by many schools. Now a party from one of those schools was striding enthusiastically towards him enjoying the bright sunshine and crisp early morning mountain air. They were led by a woman wearing stout walking shoes and of equally stout proportions herself and behind her was a raggle-taggle party of about 15 pupils, all girls. "Good morning" she called, with robust voice and a spirited cheerful wave, as if finding naked men in freezing mountain streams at the crack of dawn was an everyday occurrence, "ggggggggood mmmmorning" he replied, through chattering teeth, resisting the temptation to offer a cheery wave back as his hands at the time were elsewhere concealing a part of his anatomy he would rather not have on public view.

Eventually the party disappeared from view and he was able to extricate himself from the icy waters and resume his return to his normal camp-site, a change of clothes, a long warm up in the local pub that opened for breakfast before earning that breakfast by keeping the rest of the clientele highly amused at the tales of his latest exploit.

He was never content, always pushing the boundaries of his own technical and physical skills. Many times he became so immersed in pushing the boundaries he would ignore his own physical safety to a point of recklessness. Years later Psychotherapists would identify a behaviour called obsessional convergence, a behaviour typical of many deeply unhappy people, especially people who are repressing sexual or gender related problems. This happens when someone, often with driven energy, focuses so much on a project in hand they fail to see the dangers they are being increasingly sucked into. Years later this would at various times put his physical health, his financial security and even his liberty at risk but now it was risking his very existence.

When he was 19 his world almost ended when he was the only one in a party of three to survive a major mountaineering accident. Whilst his body healed quickly the mental pain was worse but there were many people who had taken David to their hearts and over the next few months he was helped to recovery and returned back to his beloved lake district.

Unlike his childhood he was now developing a sense of gregarious lifestyle. The loss he had suffered had somehow placed his quest for solitude into the history folder. The need to be with people, to be part of a team, was now becoming a strong desire that was replacing his need for solitude. It may just of been a growing confidence inside, a realisation that he was now good enough to take his place alongside others in society, it may have been a feeling, following that accident that killed his friends, a realisation of how vulnerable he was when so alone, whatever it was he was beginning to actually enjoy being with people as long as he always had that occasional safety net to escape into solitude.

Out of another tragic circumstance the opportunity to be part of a team and to work with people was to present itself. As part of the mountain rescue team he was called to the scene of a dreadful incident that had cost five people their lives. Working at an exhausting pace through the night in foul weather conditions they had extricated the bodies of the dead and rescued the survivors and it was an exhausted and sombre collection of people that huddled together in the weak morning daylight sipping warm drinks and making preparations to depart the grisly scene.

Many of the people he had worked with were strangers to him but he had quickly become impressed by their high level of competence and professionalism and was particularly struck by the outstanding levels of stamina and endurance they all seemed to possess. Now, talking with them for the first time in more relaxed circumstances he was to discover the admiration was mutual and they had in turn noticed how he had managed to reach right inside himself to find those extra reserves of energy and strength. These people revealed that they were a team of instructors from a centre that specialised in field craft and survival skills and they were always on the lookout for other potential outdoor and physical pursuit's instructors. After a casual conversation that to David appeared to take on the nature of a job interview centre he was finally persuaded to apply for a place on a residential instructor's course in Wales before returning back "home."

Most of the training, based in the Brecon beacons, consisted of wilderness survival, orienteering and quite brutal stamina building. Night navigation was a must. Eventually the climax of the survival training was reached, being dropped in the middle of nowhere, no food, just 1 litre of water, a map, compass and a list of way points. For three days they were to survive, navigate a 100km route over wild untracked terrain reporting into way points each day, but otherwise have no contact with civilisation whatsoever. To make it serious, as if it needed any more difficulty involved, they were told that whilst they would be tracked they must avoid all contact, being frequently "captured" would count towards probable disqualification.

One at a time each candidate was dropped off in the bleak featureless terrain. For three days the only contact each candidate was likely to have was at each waypoint at the end of each day or each time the "tracking teams" were to "find and paint" them. For most it was a daunting prospect, facing for what to them was the most arduous challenge of their lives whilst completely cast adrift from any safety net. For David, who as a child often sought solitary comfort from his internal pain by hiding away from civilisation, who as an adult resorted to long solo treks across uncharted high mountain terrain to find that solitary exclusion, this was to be food and drink.

No one saw him again until the end of the exercise. No tracking team ever found him. None of the "friendly" farmers recruited as "spotters" were to ever see him. He avoided all contact at waypoints just leaving sign that he had been there. The "game" became more serious, the efforts to find him grew, the challenge to find him and the frustration of not being able to often produced even anger. These feelings that were to be felt by the Instructors increased with the passing of every day and almost by the hour but the first they were to see of him was three days later wandering cheerfully along the reservoir road towards the rendezvous point at the end of the exercise. He was also spot on time, arriving at the exact start time of the two hour finishing period.

He, like all the others, had clearly suffered. His arms and legs were a mass of bruises and sores from falls and stumbles caused by the need for rapid progress over difficult terrain, often in darkness and with extreme tiredness adding to the hazards. His socks were blood- soaked from feet blistered and cut to pieces, his clothing soaked and covered in mud but it still didn't stop his lips and mouth moving together in harmony to issue the usual provocative challenge, not a wise thing with which to greet people nursing wounded pride and bruised egos!

It was a "no win – no lose" situation for him. In not physically showing his presence by reporting into the waypoints he had broken all the rules. His combatively aggressive attitude to some of the training staff had won him few friends but there was on the other hand glowing, if grudging, admiration for the skills and endurance he had shown. The bad boy managed to make good again, he was voted top candidate at the end of this part of the training.

However it was also necessary to obtain a qualification in white water canoeing. Something everyone was assured he was capable of as it would appear listening to him, when he enthusiastically went in front of the initial selection committee, his canoeing skills were only matched by his mountaineering ones. They were to soon find His legendary skills as a canoeist owed more to a fertile imagination and a sense of theatrical exaggeration than they did to anything somewhat more practical.

The course was being held at a location between Hereford and Ross on Wye a few miles above the lower river Wye where it enters a series of gorges known as Symonds Yat. It was tidal and heavy rains had ensured it was in flood with a fast current flowing. After a few days practicing manoeuvres, which in David's case largely consisted of learning a variety of techniques for righting an upturned canoe, it was time for the first major test, a 20 mile trip down to a location just north of the small hamlet of Tintern.

All went well at the beginning, which for David meant he had actually pushed off from the shore in an upright plane and still afloat rather than the customary "upside down, head in the water" plane, and made good progress towards the destination.

A few hundred yards from Tintern disaster struck. He lost his paddle. Now, only able to ensure his canoe stayed reasonably upright he hurtled south on the racing currents. At Tintern the receiving crews from the training centre waited in anticipation, then with excitement spotted his tiny craft approaching, were slightly perturbed as they noticed it was approaching at a speed just a little less than that of a low flying jet fighter before becoming totally alarmed as it sped past the waiting onlookers on its way to the Bristol channel and ultimately the open sea.

Jumping into every available road vehicle the waiting onlookers, now turned rescue team, hurtled off down the river bank road trying to keep in visual contact with the runaway craft and its rather alarmed occupant. David knew it was soon to approach the series of mud flats, ox-bow loops and whirlpools known as Wyntours leap. He attempted to organise some form of steerage by various gyrations of his body wedged into the cramped craft and had managed to get closer to the bank and in a slower current. Ahead was a patch of trees and with one last effort he managed to stretch and grab hold of a branch. The craft violently tried to turn on itself nearly wrenching his arms out of their sockets, went dangerously broadside to the current, twisted again causing him to lose his grip and with a jerk launched itself forward before with a shuddering jolt coming to a halt deeply impaled into a mud flat.

He sat there, breathless, mind whirling, pulse racing whilst 200 feet above him onlookers started to line the cliff edge. As he looked up he could make out the pale and worried faces of his back-up team, fellow classmates, just about everyone from the school who had been pressed into taking part in an impromptu rescue attempt. Determined to show all was well and really it was just one of those things that are nonchalantly shrugged off he struggled out of the canoe, stood precariously on an exposed tree root and with a jaunty wave to the relieved onlookers jauntily leapt onto dry land before less than jauntily sinking waist deep into stinking horrible glutinous mud.

There were more adventures to follow but by brute determination, a bit of luck and a near case of terminal heart failure for every instructor he worked with he eventually gained all qualifications necessary and returned back to the training centre to spend a 6 month period working as a mountaineering and outdoor survival instructor.

Most of the residents of the school were young people that were from backgrounds that in any other place would be called tough. Most on arriving at the centre realised from the beginning that they had yet to find out what the word meant. These were young men, often from backgrounds of growing up from tough inner city areas, many with backgrounds of approved schools and borstals, who formed the majority. These were people who as children had grown up often with learning difficulties, children from broken homes, children with behavioural difficulties, children who were just "different".

He had a close affinity with them and could empathise with their problems. He soon learned how to spot the bullies and bringing them down to earth in a hard and potentially hazardous regime of rock climbing, canoeing, orienteering and trekking over harsh mountainous terrain was not difficult. He was able to communicate with the most reserved and withdrawn boy, to reach inside that child and encourage him to find confidence and belief from within; he would spend hours each night helping boys often with severe learning difficulties, write letters home. Someone who only a few years earlier was himself taken away from home, friends and family because he was "different" was able to reach across those boundaries of "adult in charge" these children kept to protect themselves and bring those boundaries down. For these children he was a natural leader, someone they could trust to see them through any ordeal, lead them safely through any hardship, someone they could call upon to help confront their most intense fears.

Working with David they learnt self-reliance, found a new confidence and become possessed of self-respect. Many would reveal, in contacts and letters written to him afterwards, how much that time spent at that school turned around their lives. For David this would only hone even further his sense of compassion and his zeal for direct intervention in the cause of that compassion.

By this time his permanent home was in Manchester having left London at the earliest opportunity to move further north and closer to the rock climbing areas of Scotland, Snowdonia and the Lake District. The intensity with which he threw himself into mountaineering was keeping the pain away, he belonged to a small close knit fraternity, he was seen as totally macho and as something he felt to be acceptable to him, his parents and society in general. Physically though this activity was taking its toll, the legacies of injury after injury were accumulating, but for now he was at the peak of physical fitness and they were to remain unnoticed for many years to come.

He also started developing other problems. For months he had been experiencing balance problems. He had always suffered from vertigo, strangely not the only prominent mountaineer of the day to have such a problem, but this was different. On a number of occasions he found himself becoming completely unnerved on even relatively easy climbs. Year later he was to suffer with violent neuralgia that brought back and magnified those balance problems. Whether this was a precursor to those later problems or not he would never know but now he was finding himself in an increasingly hazardous position. The obsessional drive to keep improving, never being satisfied, was still driving him forward into ever more risky exploits but now these risks were manifestly increased.

It was not just climbing upwards that was being seriously compromised. On one occasion he had travelled for a weekend's climbing in North Wales. Having completed a climb of exhausting difficulty as it was approaching nightfall he started to descend via a gulley of very moderate difficulty. Half way down he found himself unable to even stand upright. Below him was a steep slope of loose boulders and jagged rocks, His head swam, his vision became blurred, his footing went out from underneath him. He arrived at the bottom of the slope in a cloud of dust and a clatter of rolling boulders. Other climbers went to his aid but he was unable to feel his legs. An ambulance was called but by the time it arrived, having to travel along narrow mountain roads, he felt feeling start to return. The ambulance team wanted to carry him to the waiting vehicle and on to hospital but with brute obstinacy he refused, insisting on trying to stand. Finally after an hour he managed a painful few steps.

He eventually managed to make it back to base camp and friends offered to drive him home but this would ruin their weekend and also David was again displaying those traits he displayed as a child of when hurt retreating inside himself, retreating into a world of isolated self-reliance. He insisted on going home, hitch-hiking all the way, his 50kg rucksack bearing down on his injured back.

It was an agonising 20 hour journey home. For days afterwards he could hardly walk, there was blood in his urine but he curled up in his lair and refused help. Slowly he healed and life returned to normal. 20 years later after being examined for spinal problems after severe muscle spasms it was discovered he had carried his 60kg pack home on a back that had been fractured, compression fractures causing a partial fusing of two vertebrae.

Throughout this macho period one thing stood out oddly as a characteristic. He seemed always to relate easier to females than males. Night after night in the hugely macho environment of the local pub the same pattern would become evident. Always the first at the bar, always the one first to relate tales of mentally demanding heroics, physical extremes and hardships, but as the pub filled up and the beer fuelled the testosterone so he would shyly retreat out of the way, spending the rest of the night in conversation with wives, girlfriends or whatever talking about everything else on the planet other than climbing or other typical male pursuits. Many expressed surprise at the sensitivity that in these times would often creep out from under the tough macho exterior but in those days it was always a source of embarrassment to him, often sparking a compensating compulsion to go off and do something even more physically extreme.

He had by this time put his faith on the back burner. Praying to God was not macho, not seen as essential in his life but looking back at the charmed life he led it is fairly obvious now to see that if he had left God for a while God

Trapped

most certainly had not left him. Meanwhile in terms of his mortal existence it was Fortunate something else was to come into his life to turn him away from this inevitable path to destruction.

His sexual orientation greatly assisted with his need to prove acceptability. The rugged macho image of a lifestyle mountaineer was attractive to many women and he felt no need to be shy about pursuing his biological sexual role!! One June, shortly after celebrating his birthday he with a few friends took themselves off to a party in Oldham. They were not invited but were all equally adept at gate-crashing such events, especially when the party was being hosted by a young attractive nurse from the local hospital and attended by a number of her equally attractive colleagues. Entering the flat where it was being held his poor eyesight needed help so a friend identified all the available "talent". At 8 o-clock was a slim girl with long brown hair, 9 o-clock was the flighty girl who had opened the door, at 10 o-clock was a tall angular girl with a bloke. It got to 12 o-clock, a curly haired slim leggy girl who it appeared was the hostess. It went no further. By 5am in the morning David knew that Jo, the tall leggy hostess, was going to be his wife. For both it was love at first sight.

Marriage was something in the distant future. Since leaving school David had worried even less about his finances than he did about his physical safety. He had no job, no qualifications, no track record in mainstream employment and before such an event could be contemplated he needed to find a precious source of funds. However marriage became a necessity when a few months into their relationship Jo announced she was pregnant. In December that year they married, he was a few months away from becoming a father, they were totally penniless and soon Jo, the sole provider of an income, was going to have to cease work. It was time to get serious about life. At this most propitious moment the climbing years was over. Becoming a father would be the final proof he needed to himself and society that he really was a Man so the mountaineering lifestyle was expendable. What he needed was to turn the clock back and just like the rest of his peer group who left school together a few years earlier he now focussed on a career and a regular income. Career number one was firmly over. Career number two was yet to begin.

Chapter 5:
The business career

CAREER number two got off to a faltering start. Finding a job was not so easy as it was when he first left school. There simply were not that many vacancies for someone with no academic or vocational qualifications whose main achievements since leaving school consisted of totally irrelevant mountaineering exploits. The urgency to find gainful employment though increased dramatically when in April, a couple of weeks before his birthday he became a father to twin boys. However there was something called the Open University, despite no academic qualifications he could still sign up and do a degree course so with what little funds he had from the odd job or two he managed to find he enrolled. For the next few months life was to be a busy father, studying for a degree and job hunting.

The job hunting he pursued in typical style. The first editions of the local newspaper, the main source of job vacancies, were first distributed in Central Manchester 9 miles away. By the time the local newspaper reached his area anyone getting the first editions would have a few hours head start so he solved it by amongst everything else walking

18 miles a day to and from Manchester City centre to be able to access the very first editions.

Their financial situation was desperate but when the boys were 10 months old Jo managed to secure a job as a warden of a sheltered residence for old people, a flat was thrown in and the small income provided a degree of refuge from mounting financial problems.

Thanks to Jo they had a breathing space but even when he found a job it often didn't last long, he was still adjusting to working in controlled environments again where he was not for the most part living on his wits, his own self-reliance, leading from the front. Following from the back and working in the front line with rules that clearly did not suit his temperament and with leaders whom he mostly regarded as second rate followers often stressed his naturally low tolerance beyond acceptable levels to him. He lost count of the number of ways the same words "you're fired" was phrased after a stormy confrontation with someone who unfortunately for David was the boss.

Eventually after a number of false starts he was offered a job with a placement agency. This agency, unlike many of its competitors, had a very slick American approach to its business insisting its "counsellors", as the staff were called, adhered to very closely controlled methods of interviewing people to be placed, employers looking for people and media looking to sell advertising space. Even the mode of dress was strictly controlled.

After a few weeks he found himself in the department that took calls from employers looking for people. One call he took was from a local branch of a French oil multinational looking for a marketing assistant. He launched himself into the standard speech outlining the terms and conditions but was cut short by a rather bored secretary at the other end saying "blah blah blah!! Heard it loads of times, could repeat it back to you, this is what we want, I know all the terms etc," He took down the details of this very attractive job and after hanging up he looked at the job description again and especially at the age and type of person this company was looking for. He looked at the salary, the job prospects, and the fringe benefits.

Taking a deep breath he rang them back and got through to the bored secretary again. "Hello, its Bill from the agency ... we have just the right person for you... he is"... "Blah Blah Blah!!" interrupted the bored secretary, "He is the perfect age, got the perfect qualifications, got the perfect background and can start right away ... heard it all before, can he come for interview tomorrow?". "Sorry, no he can't" replied David, "he is free now though but in so much demand, by tomorrow he will probably be snapped up, he can come round now" A pause on the other end as bored secretary consulted her boss, then "Ok, next 10 minutes, what's his name?" "David" said David, and "He's on his way now"

The boss finished reading the application form. He was large aggressive person who pulled no punches when it came to interviewing but David gave as good as he got and it had been a lively and vigorous interview. . "So", boomed the boss, "It says here you are working at the moment but doesn't say who for"?

David gave the name of the placement agency. "No, the boss said in a rather bored tone, "Not who sent you, who are you working for now?" David took a deep breath, and repeated his answer. The boss sighed, then in a "Watch my lips" tone of voice asked again who David worked for. David repeated the name of the placement agency.

The boss stared, the penny dropped, the stare intensified, and then he threw back his head and roared with laughter. "And I suppose" he said, "your role in this company is to call people like my secretary back and tell her you have an unbelievably perfect person for us who must be interviewed straight away before being snapped up by someone else?" David gulped out an affirmative reply. "And when can this unbelievably perfect person for us be available to join us" snapped out the boss. "Probably about ten minutes after going back and telling the company what I've been up to" replied David. The boss roared with laughter again, then said "This afternoon I'm too busy, tomorrow morning?"

He had joined the marketing department wanting to be a salesman but they had other ideas. The manager he worked with had identified a sharp analytical mind with high numeric skills and he was encouraged to apply for a position with the corporate financial management department which he did and was soon rewarded with his first upward career move.

Now he could throw himself into his new career, in between being a father and studying for his degree he would with driven energy throw himself into project after project, so much so he was often counselled by senior management that he should give himself a break, ease off a bit, or else he would burn out. As well as this wise counselling they also showed their faith in him by agreeing to sponsor his Open University course, a welcome release as the historic accumulation of loans and unpaid bills was creating severe financial hardship.

It was just in time for there was an incident a few weeks earlier that had threatened to unleash the repressed Gender Dysphoria and send him back into that deeply unhappy world of confusion and dislocation he felt as a child. Jo had been poisoned, a severe form of food poisoning and was in an isolation wing of a specialist hospital for six weeks. During this time, for the first time in his memory, David felt a very deep desire to dress in Jo's clothes. Psychiatrists would later identify in his brain very strong nurturing instincts and recognise this incident as a deep desire to take over the mother role to his infant children but for him it was deeply disturbing, after all, he was not just a bloke, he was a very macho tough mountaineer of a bloke and blokes like that simply do not have leanings towards cross dressing.

Shortly after being awarded his degree David was approached by an American multinational that had recently acquired a British manufacturing company in a nearby town. He had been recommended to them by a partner in a placement agency and after being invited for an interview he was made an offer he couldn't refuse. It was a propitious moment. A year earlier the world had been gripped by an oil supply crisis, the oil supply industry was in difficulties and David's job was under threat.

This company had sponsored places with a prestigious UK business school and he was offered a place to study for an external Masters Degree in Business Administration, an opportunity he grabbed with both hands for not only was it a significant career opportunity it would again give him something to immerse himself in when not working or being a father and husband.

He had only just settled himself into this job when he was again approached, this time by an ailing British Manufacturer. They offered him a senior financial management position with a highly attractive remuneration package including subsidising his studies for an MBA. It was an offer he couldn't refuse.

There was plenty to do at this company. Like many companies involved in manufacturing this was the time of a major reconstruction. The financial planning department which he was initially recruited into was massive, it needed to be. This company liked to produce business plans, for three months a vast army of financial managers would beaver away producing the annual corporate plan which, often through coercion, and sometimes intimidation, from operational management, would be a document forecasting future profits of staggering proportions. Unfortunately by the time it had been reviewed through the various levels of senior management it would be redundant, looming reality suggesting the optimistic forecasts of billions of pound profits were hopelessly exaggerated so revision after downward revision was needed to achieve something slightly more compatible with reality. However by the time that the final finished result was published it was also just in time for the forecasts of now modest profits to be seen as also wildly optimistic and a recovery plan needed to avert the even more obvious reality of looming mega losses. David soon revived his childhood skills of writing dreamy fairy tale nonsense prose and which was widely applauded by senior financial management as the nearest anyone ever got to reality.

Soon something else gave him the opportunity to attract the attention of senior management. A small subsidiary company had dramatically lost its head of finance right in the middle of the planning cycle and David was hastily dropped in to produce at short notice a business plan for the forthcoming company wide review. For someone like David this opportunity was perfect for to meet the planning deadlines he had to throw himself into working around the clock with forceful energy. The plan he produced was a masterpiece of hard-headed business reality unlike the fanciful projections of submissions from other parts of the organisation. Under his financial management this company in the next few months was to be the only subsidiary to achieve results that were actually planned for.

One of the first moves he made in restoring the fortunes of this ailing company was to re-organise the sprawling accounts and financial management departments. In doing this he astounded everyone by appointing as a new head of the costing department a total outsider bypassing a whole line-up of candidates who considered themselves to be the natural replacement leaders. It wasn't appointing an outsider that shocked everyone though, it was the fact this outsider was a woman. For the first time he demonstrated a trait that would be a mark of his business management, his implicit faith in female professional managers and advisers that he demonstrated by appointing them into positions that had previously been considered all male domains.

For the next few years his progress up the career ladder was steadily rapid. Having turned round the fortunes of one ailing company he was dropped into another, larger one to do the same again. Very often the terms of reference was either "sort it or shut it" and he developed a two fold reputation, either that of a manager who could restore to health the fortunes of a sick company or someone who would move decisively to cut the losses if he felt a business had reached the point of no return. His reputation as a "Sort it or shut it" manager blossomed and after each successful turn around he would be sent on another mission, each time the challenges getting bigger and more intense.

His reputation may of grown hugely but the price paid for him and his family was also huge. Jo hardly saw her husband or the children their father, working away or working all hours, no time for holidays, intense and serious when at home, often working and worst of all three house moves in that time. It was a 120 hour working week running at 120 miles an hour existence. It was again that distinctive pattern of behaviour of always pushing the boundaries, pushing himself to exhaustion, never seeing when a commitment had moved beyond the achievable to the physically and mentally exhausting barely possible.

It was not all work though. One of their moves had taken them to a small village where many people were like themselves, working parents bringing up young children. It was a highly gregarious existence, many friendships being forged by the common factor of children attending the same school. However not all the families raising young children were completely functional. At the edge of the village living in two caravans parked on farming land was a large extended family. A common sight around the village was the eldest child of this family, a young girl called Maria, pushing the youngest child, her baby sister, in a pushchair. This young girl had a bit of a roguish reputation, the lids on local sweet jars being nailed down when she approached, but to David she was always a pleasant, well mannered child with an endearing smile and if her clothes were rags they were at least clean rags.

Then as this girl approached her teenage years she began to change. Her skin pallor grew pale, her eyes took on a haunted look and the engaging smile was less present. David, like many, mostly female, members of their social group expressed concern. One day the police arrived, Maria's Father and Uncle were arrested; she was taken off into care. She had been suffering from sexual abuse and exploitation. Many men in the village voiced their desire to tear the two molesters apart limb by limb but David just cried, privately hiding those feminine tears. Inside him their was an anger, an anger that would never go away and would in later years help fuel a crusade against child abuse. His anger though was at himself. He had anger that he saw the suffering in this child's eyes, had suspicions but did nothing. He harboured anger that this beautiful child was so despoiled, anger that she had been so hurt, all he wanted to do was to cry for her. Her haunted eyes would be an image that would in turn haunt him for years to come.

As usual whenever he showed feminine feelings, allowed himself to display typical feminine traits, he compensated by finding very male things to do. He was now working at the head office of this multinational and this company had a number of works football teams one of which played in a semi-professional league. Even though he had not kicked a football in a serious way since being at school he joined one of their football teams.

Trapped

It couldn't be the Sunday league side pottering out on the football field the Sunday morning after the night before though. He had to be with the best. Running a minimum of 5 miles every night over the hilly terrain surrounding the town this head office was located in he brought his fitness levels up. He would attend every training session going. He started to move through the teams, from Sunday league to third reserves, to first reserves, to a couple of outings with the senior side until eventually a regular first team choice for the senior team playing in a semi-professional league.

It was not long though before injuries started to take their toll. Those joints so damaged from the climbing years would swell up just from the training, he would play match after competitive match with knee and ankle joints almost permanently swollen, supporting elastic bandages holding everything in place and a diet of pain-killers keeping the pain at bay. Eventually one tackle too many, a visit to the local hospital, torn cartilage the diagnosis and his football career was over.

So almost was his career with this company. He was to make one of the most dramatic decisions of his life, to give up a lucrative and safe contract, his job, cars, and status and risk everything joining a management team of a state owned company that was being broken up into small pieces and sold off. He had been approached by the manager of this small subsidiary and a 10 minute chat in a pub and David knew he had met a like-minded soul, someone with the same ambition, the same ideas, and the same views on becoming the biggest and best. David also felt, and was never to be proved wrong, he had met someone of the highest personal integrity and someone whom he could trust completely.

He had no hesitation in saying yes to the invitation. With no guarantees of success of the venture he as finance director prepared and orchestrated the management buyout. His initial instincts regarding the person he had that 10 minute chat with, the person who was to be chairman of the new company, proved to be justified over and over again. He was working with someone whom he could have total respect for, someone as committed as he was to making the company grow and one of the few people he had met in his life whose ambitions would match his own. They were to be highly successful and acquisition after acquisition followed. In the next two years the company grew 20 times its original size.

Now, responsible only to the chairman and with unlimited scope for his driven energy that obsessional convergence was unrestrained, the pace grew more driven, the dangers to his health of always being on the move, eating lunch and dinner on the go, dashing from one meeting to another, never resting, never reflecting, was ignored.

He had started getting attacks of neuralgia, a searing pain behind the eyes and down the face shortly after throwing himself into his latest project. They increased in intensity, duration and frequency. The pain was unbearable but still he ignored it, totally focussed on the business in hand. Finally one day it snapped out of control, after 24 hours of severe unrelenting pain he finally had to seek medical help. He saw a specialist, was rushed into hospital and for the next four weeks was given a whole battery of tests.

The doctors were mystified. Everything pointed to a close cousin of migraine called cluster headache. However cluster headache was not normally found in people with migraine and David had been a chronic migraine sufferer for most of his life. Cluster headache was normally episodic but this had deteriorated into an unrelenting chronic condition. Episodes of cluster headache can last up to 40 minutes; David was having attacks lasting for hours. Worse there were signs of increasing interruption to neural activity, leg and arm muscles on one side were significantly weakened.

Trapped

There was no way he could carry on working. The condition was out of control. It was going to take every ounce of the strength and willpower he had left just to survive. Psychiatrists would later say it could well of been an auto-immune reaction, as his body weakened due to exhaustion so the internal unhappiness caused a reaction.

Whatever the fundamental cause at the age of 41 his health was broken. He was retired. He was financially secure. The company chairman, the same person that a couple of years earlier he had such warm feelings towards, displayed that characteristic integrity and honesty and rewarded David with generous compensation for having to leave so abruptly and in other ways made it his business to ensure that David was to be financially secure. Yet another person in his life that David would be eternally grateful to, and not without a lot of love for as well. Career number two was firmly over and it was to be a long time before career number three could begin. For now it was to be survival and recovery that the manic driven energy was to be focussed upon.

Chapter 6:
Recovery

His life was shattered. It was the psychological equivalent of a 120mph express train slamming into a brick wall. With nothing to focus his mind on again all those feelings of being ill at ease with whom he was, being incomplete and inadequate, of being different resurfaced. To a degree these would have been normal feelings with many people who had suffered such a physical breakdown but this was someone who by every measure had been brilliantly successful, satisfied all the macho criteria of being aggressive and logically ruthless and such intense feelings of profound discomfort and failure to associate in a male sense would be strangely at odds with this background of success.

He had been referred onwards by the local specialists to the National Neurological Hospital in London where his treatment was being seen by a specialist of international renown. The illness continued unabated and to some extent he was used as a guinea pig, not only recounting episodes of neuralgia on video to be used as a teaching tool for other specialists around the world but also being given different cocktails of new drugs, some of which in turn had side

Jennifer Brown

effects that made him quite ill. Through all of this he still needed to find distraction to the feelings emerging from within and in the autumn of 1989 it happened.

He was watching a television programme made by Jon Pilger, a well known and well respected investigative journalist on amongst other things Indo China and human rights. Jon was explaining how ten years after one of the worst genocides in recorded history had been perpetrated on the people of Cambodia by the Khmer Rouge, who had seized power in 1975 following the collapse of the American involvement in the Vietnamese war; it was the Khmer Rouge that still represented those people in the international lobby of the United Nations. Pilger went on to explain how the Khmer Rouge had been ousted by the Vietnamese in 1978 who then imposed their own puppet government on the people but despite the outrage of the killing fields as the United States had still not recovered from defeat by the Vietnamese it refused to recognise this government or allow it to represent the people in the UN, an action endorsed by fellow security council member The United Kingdom. Having brought this to the attention of the people Pilger closed the programme by exhorting viewers to write to their members of Parliament.

David did. He did not stop there though. He wrote to every single MP, all 650 of them. He wrote to every single member of the House of Lords. He wrote to the Queen and to the president of the United States.

Within days replies started to flow back, and as replies to replies started to fuel the mail flow a trickle turned into a flood. By the end of two weeks he had sent out over 1,500 letters. The furore he caused had forced an emergency debate in the House of Commons; just one private individual had sparked a national debate but it was to go even further than just a national issue. That debate was to have repercussions that spilled over to the other side of the Atlantic and eventually to the United Nations itself.

The opposition spokesperson in her opening address to parliament quoted his original letter. Aid charities became involved, unable to involve themselves in politics they were glad of finding someone to fire their bullets, the argument spilled over to the other side of the Atlantic and a stream of international correspondence added to the torrent of mail arriving and leaving. There were also more sinister developments. Parcels started arriving in the middle of the night, delivered mysteriously by hand, just left leaning by the front door, containing amongst other things leaked memo's of meetings and suppressed copies of international relief reports on Cambodia.

At this point most people would of considered enough was enough, getting into the arena of international politics involving such a sensitive geo-political region had risks associated with it that would of deterred practically anyone but that obsessional trait so distinctive of his way of repressing Gender Dysphoria took over. Totally oblivious of the dangers it was leading him into he pushed himself into making further efforts to influence change for good.

Suddenly the mail, which by then had reduced from the initial flood to a steady trickle of around 20 letters a day stopped. A few days later the mail for the previous few days would arrive in bulk then cease for another few days, the cycle repeating over and over again. There would be a pause on the telephone before voice contact was made. The strangest incident though was the blue ford car that would park by the side of the road about 100 yards away. There was no need for anyone to park there, it was a rural secondary road, his house had only a couple of neighbours either side, and to front and back were empty fields. One day David left the house but walked in the opposite direction before crossing the road, going into a field and walking back along a footpath that skirted the road before re-entering behind this car.

Walking back to the car he was just in time to see the passenger packing away what looked to be a camera. The driver had is window opened as David passed so he could not resist making confrontational contact. "Cup of tea chaps, must be boring spying on your own citizens". Without a word being said the window was raised, the car driven off and it was never to be seen there again.

No one will ever know who they were or what was going on. It is almost certain that obsessional convergence had caused him to be oblivious to the danger he was walking in to and either legal or other lines were crossed. This would not be the last time. 14 years later it would happen again with far more devastating consequences. As it was the situation in Cambodia had entered a stage where serious debate was now being held amongst the international community and a few years later the Khmer Rouge representation in the UN would be replaced by something more representative of the people. His involvement was reaching a natural and fortuitously timely end.

There was a sad sequel to this story. In "the killing fields", the much acclaimed film that chronicled the genocide in Cambodia, the part of Dith Pran, the Cambodian assistant to American journalists who 's story of escape the film revolved around was played by Haing Ngor, A doctor at the time who's family were mostly murdered and who himself suffered so much. Years later David was invited to meet him in his new home in Los Angeles but on the eve of flying there he learnt the awful news that Haing Ngor had been murdered, allegedly by a Vietnamese criminal gang he was investigating..

The cerebral-vascular spasms were getting no better and leg and arm muscles were still weak. Doctors recommended he take up walking for regular exercise. He did, From Lands end to John O'Groats. He had always been fascinated about walking this route and for months pored over every possible

Trapped

route variant plotting in the tiniest detail the maximum avoidance of major roads. Jo had elected to walk it with him, Adam, one of their Son's was co-opted as the sole back up team hauling everything in a huge motor home. In 1990 they set off and 63 days and over 1,000 miles later arrived at John O'Groats having walked through dreadful weather and with David being beset by frequent episodes of illness and drug-induced fatigue to leg muscles. It was a monumental achievement, three people, Jo who hated walking, Adam, himself with learning difficulties, navigating the length of the country driving a 2 ton large motor home along some tiny country lanes to places almost inaccessible to road vehicles of any size and David struggling with a chronic debilitating illness and hampered by drugs producing highly unpleasant and unwanted side effects.

It would have been enough of an achievement for anyone but not for David. The following evening after their arrival they were sat in a café at Wick, a few miles from their point of triumphant arrival a couple of days before, and were starting the long laborious journey home. The café was shared with another party, young adults whose behaviour made them stand out. They were adults suffering with Downs Syndrome. They all had severe learning and social difficulties and some were severely physically handicapped. It made him realise just what gifts he had in life, that whatever his problems there were always others he could reach out to and help.

Returning home he explained his plan to Jo. On the anniversary of their arrival at John O'Groats set off on the return journey, walking from North to South, only make it a fund raising event to help a college who provided residential help to young people with severe physical difficulties, young people who would never be able to accomplish the physical feats David had felt to be so blessed in being given the opportunity to do. After a lot of heart-searching Jo agreed. With both of them there had been a feeling of anti-climax arriving at John O'Groats; this would be the opportunity to close the chapter and to give to others so desperately less fortunate.

The following year they did the return journey, throwing in for fun an extra 40 miles to include Dunnett head and Lizard Point, the true most northerly and Southerly geographical points of Mainland Great Britain, 1067 miles this time in 43 days.

The fund-raising was approached with the same energy as the walking. The collection boxes that were always carried were shaken under thousands of noses. Article after article was written detailing their exploits and published into whatever media could be harassed into providing print space. Back home talk after talk was given to organisation after organisation.

The winter season of talks had now become the spring season of talks. One of the talks was to a local round table. They were an affable bunch and David, his gregarious self beginning to show, was enjoying a pre-dinner drink in the bar with a few of them. Attendance for dinner was called, they trooped upstairs, pint glasses in hand, and a very affable dinner followed with the usual compliment of after dinner drinks. Finally he was introduced and with another freshly poured pint in front of him stood up to address the throng with another blockbusting, earth moving, rousing speech guaranteed to force the emptying of pockets of even the most hard-hearted scrooge.

Finishing his speech he sat down to thunderous applause from the handful of people who had managed to stay awake and refreshed himself by draining his pint glass which was dutifully and generously refilled. A question and answer session was then announced. He rose to his feet, somewhat unsteadily, to answer one question, a genteel sip from his glass, someone rushing off to refill the drained dry glass, another question, another genteel sip, another refill, the questions focussed on what he will do next, will he ever want to emulate those feats again, what was to follow, was this the last time?

Somewhat hazily he replied, mumbling something about twice being enough for anyone, only an obsessive fool would do it a third time, what did they think he was, some form of driven idiot that did not know when to stop?. At least that's what he thought he had said. Finally the evening ended. He had been most warmly received. It was time to make his way shakily home for the following day he and Jo were going on holiday for 10 days to sunny Italy.

Returning from holiday duly refreshed he was somewhat perplexed when a visitor called and in the middle of explaining how they had missed some awful weather managed to express surprise that after the awful weather of last year she was surprised that David would contemplate repeating the same walk again. A phone caller that evening expressed in passing he thought David must be mad. Tuesday the local newspaper rang, they wanted to write a story on "third again". They kindly sent David a copy of the edition of their newspaper printed a couple of weeks earlier whilst the couple were on holiday in Italy. There, prominently carried on the inside front page, beneath block headlines of "Marathon walker sets off again" was a story detailing how at a fundraising dinner that weekend, just before leaving for a "business trip" to Italy, David had used the event to declare to the surprise of the world in general and in greater surprise to himself in particular he was setting off again that Summer.

He agonised over the predicament he found himself in. He was totally unprepared, unfit and unwell as the neuralgia continued to hammer his body. He had no planning in place although his Son Steven had volunteered to act as back up volunteering six weeks of his own study time to do so. There was no way he could face the boredom of doing the same trip again along the same route so a whole new schedule and route would have to be devised. Finally, feeling himself unable to say no, or to retract, he set out to do it again, although Jo had had enough, she wisely stayed sat home.

He had to push the boundaries, 1,020 miles in 35 days, those 35 days including 5 days of inactivity due to illness and injury, his son Steven, towing a caravan, acting as back-up. Whatever the circumstances may of been, a new route, a lack of planning, a lack of fitness and still beset my health problems all meant no difference, whatever happened it just had to be better than the times before.

The first injury was ominous. 100 miles from John O'Groats his ankles started to stiffen and swell. Just before the Mountain resort town of Aviemore the pain had reached excruciating levels and walking had become almost impossible. Slumping against the door of a café he fumbled for his mobile phone to ring Steven. It just was not his day. The café door opened inwards and a customer wanted to leave. As she pulled open the door she was startled to find falling into her arms was a box-rattling charity walker clutching a mobile phone. Stepping smartly to one side she allowed this charity walker to fall to the floor with a crash, box flying in one direction and phone in the other. He had no need to ring Steven, the café owner instead rang for an ambulance, only too eager to be rid of his unwanted guest.

Sinovitis, a precursor to arthritis, was the diagnosis. He was given a strong dose of pain killers, a prescription for a weeks supply, patched up with anti-inflammatory tablets and creams and told to rest up for a minimum of seven days or risk permanent damage. He rested for two. Then on the third day, as anti-inflammatory drugs started to work and pain killers masked the pain, he set off again. Being still, resting, having nothing to do but think and reflect, was not something his mind would allow.

He limped on through Scotland and most of England, teeth gritted against the pain from his creaking ankles and

Trapped

screaming Neuralgia coursing down his face. Into Devon and soon the bulk of Dartmoor was looming in front. The challenge of going over, not round, was too much. The weather was glorious, dry and warm, why not?

Crossing over a shoulder of Dartmoor from near the small town of Okehampton and disaster nearly struck. He was beset by a sudden and intense bout of neuralgia. Within five minutes parts of his face and left eye felt as though they were on fire. His vision seriously reduced from watering eyes, themselves screwed up in pain, he could scarcely see where his feet were going. Desperate to find shelter from the bright sunshine he scanned the map for the quickest way to the road, where he at least might be able to summon help from his son. Choosing a route that followed a rough and steep track he set off down but lost his footing half way. His knee twisted over with a sickening wrench. Now, hardly able to bear any weight on his injured leg, with pain screaming down his face, he was in a perilous predicament.

It was a slow agonising descent. Every step had to be deliberate, one more fall and his chances of reaching the road unaided would disappear, he had no signal for his mobile phone and his son had no idea he had chosen to go off the road route planned and instead was in the wilds of Dartmoor. Finally he made it to the road and in excruciating pain managed to hobble half a mile to a welcome pub.

The landlady of the pub couldn't of done more, fetching towels soaked in ice water, making compresses from more crushed ice and ringing Steven who arrived in rapid time armed with handfuls of anti-inflammatory tablets and pain killers. Eventually he managed to make it back to the caravan and spent an anxious evening and sleepless night trying to work miracles on a badly swollen knee.

Despite everything giving up was not in the itinerary. The next few days he limped on, the swellings started to subside, his pace quickened. He eventually reached Lands

End in record time but with ankle and knee joints that would never again support such an effort. They had signalled they had, quite literally, come to the end of the road.

As always again he had obsessively pushed those boundaries to the point of over-commitment. In his climbing years it was his life he risked, in his business years his marriage and physical heath, over Cambodia his legal safety, now it was his physical health that was again to take the toll. The accumulation of physical damage caused by the injuries sustained in his climbing years, the obsessively focussed football playing and now this marathon walking was turning ankles and knees into aching arthritic lumps. He was suffering recurrent seizures and spasms in his back muscles that had been so damaged by compensating for the compression fractures he had suffered in that climbing fall many years earlier.

Despite all these emerging problems the following year he decided to move off tarmac and walk the 630 miles of the South West Coast Path, Britain's longest and most rugged trail. Enough of a challenge in itself but he decided he was going to have no back up team, relying instead on camping and carrying everything he needed in a huge rucksack.

Again he had over committed, pushed the boundaries too far. Within a hundred miles a heavy fall had twisted those knee joints; a further fall in Cornwall during torrential downpour miles from shelter had aggravated those old spinal injuries. His ankles were swollen to the size of footballs. He carried on for another 350 miles but finally, desperate with neuralgic pain, ankle, knee and back injuries causing him excruciating joint pain and numbing sciatic pain down his legs, he was forced him to stop only 90 miles from the end. This was the end of this type of physical exploit; he had pushed too hard too far. He still needed distractions though. It was time to think about career number three.

Chapter 7:
Back to business

He could now no longer seek distraction via physical means. During these marathon walks he had written a series of articles to be published in various magazines. He now combined all the articles of the first two walks into a full length book, his first published work. Writing had now resurfaced as a major passion, his other passions of Military history and travelling to different places he decided could be combined into a tour company, one specialising in military history tours of unusual nature with small-book length explanatory brochures giving easy to read historical backgrounds to places on route. Writing was to be career number three.

It was to be as much hobby as business but to David there was no such thing as recreational pleasure; it had to be 120 mile an hour 120 hours a week distraction.

First guides to be written were modest affairs, Short 4 day walking tours to the historic centre of Rome and the defensive lines of Torres Vedras in Portugal. The driven, never content churnings inside him could not stop things there. Next, building on tours of Torres Vedras was to be a whole series of guide books covering Wellingtons campaigns in the Iberian peninsular during the Napoleonic wars. Soon 4 day tours became 7 day tours which then stretched to 10 days as the scope was widened and now itineraries stretched from Lisbon harbour through Portugal and the length of Spain to the French border.

Of course this restless, continuous charge through Latin Europe was not enough. He decided that as he was spending so much time in Italy he should at least learn to speak the language so he enrolled at a language school in Florence. This sojourn though was only a daytime activity; he needed to occupy himself at night so he also enrolled at a cooking school. Nothing in Italian cooking is done without wine, either wine poured into the food, wine poured into the chef or both and often in David's case it was both with a large part of the both ending up in the chef. His taste for wine was finding a natural home in Italy.

The large established tour company back home in England which David had negotiated a collaborative marketing deal with were being inundated with tour itineraries. It should of stopped there but the restless agitation burning away inside him forced him to seek ever more broader and challenging horizons and the United States beckoned.

In the early 90's, long before it became in general use, David had discovered the internet. He used an internet provider called CompuServe which was also very much an online community with many discussion forums. He took part with others, mostly from the United States, in such subjects as military history, political discussions and emotional support. In one of these emotional support forums he had impressed many people with his open-hearted compassion and had been encouraged to take part as a supporter and listener in a restricted access group specialising in offering emotional support to adult victims of abuse, predominantly adult survivors of child sexual abuse and domestic violence and rape. He had, after some reluctance, joined them and now was a valued member of that community, many female members acknowledging he was the first man they felt they could talk to. Through all of these activities there were many people who would be very pleased to meet him, an added incentive to providing tours across the USA.

His first focus of interest was the Civil War battlefields. Conventional tours focussed on short narratives of what happened in each location and artefacts still on show. Not good enough for someone so driven as David. The tours had to be of campaigns, following great commanders such as Lee, Grant and Sherman, from one great battlefield to another, the guides being almost full book size. For months he criss-crossed the continent, coming within an inch of being bitten by rattlesnakes in the New Mexico desert, swept away by tornado's in North Carolina, risking rising flood waters in South Carolina and sometimes driving up to 800 miles a day.

The result was a tour itinerary and a set of guides that today is still used by many tourist authorities as an "off the beaten track" guide to what really went on. He could relax, rest on his laurels, but for that driving agitation and lack of contentment inside. Something bigger and more challenging had to be there and it was,

In the early 1840's a westward expansion of the United States resulted in a trickle of pioneers crossing the continent to establish a new life on the west coast. This trickle turned into the greatest migration of peoples in modern times resulting in what became known as the Oregon Trail, and when gold was discovered, the California gold rush trails, and as the railways moved west the cattle trails such as the Santa Fe trail.

There was no break from the exhaustion and pace of writing the Civil War guides. As they finished so drafting the emigrant trails took over. Criss- crossing the mountains, risking often being trapped in snowfalls, ignoring avalanche warnings and rattlesnake warnings the result was a finite 120 page guide to the 2,200 mile Oregon trail that is still a valid and authorative work today.

Of course it could not stop there. First it was tour guides that covered half a city, then half a country, then 3 states of the United States then half a continent. The best was yet to come.

Over the years he had made many friends and had many contacts in the US military. One suggested that with the right references he could get him a trip on a US military passenger flight to Midway Island, then solely a US Military base. The thought of this electrified him for as an amateur military historian he had been fascinated by the battle of Midway, one of the greatest naval battles of all time and a pivotal battle in the second world war. The only problem was one of Distance. Midway lies in the middle of the vast Pacific ocean 6 and a half hours flight away from Hawaii which itself was 5 ½ hours flight away from Mainland United States. This did not deter David though. An idea had grown in his head and nothing was going to deter him putting it together into fruition.

Over the next few weeks he criss-crossed the pacific going to various remote and exotic places such as the Solomon Islands, Guam and Tinian. Hawaii almost became home. Finally it was ready. A tour itinerary planned over two weeks covering the 2nd World War in the Pacific. Starting with Pear Harbour, featuring the battle of Midway, the battles for the pacific Islands and finishing where the American bombers took off to deliver their atomic bombs. Only political sensitivity prevented him from including the peace park in Hiroshima as a final destination. It was a tour-de-force, and his tours, hitherto stretching to half a continent now took in half the globe. Not surprisingly when he published this tour his collaborators treated it almost as a joke but the rights to it were immediately snapped up by a United States tour company who found it to be a sell out.

By now the obsessive energy had again driven him again into over commitments. He had ignored his wife, his health, his family and almost the United States Government as he had infringed their residency laws.

Cluster headache was also re-emerging. Not as severe as it was in 1988, not as debilitating but enough of a warning signal that his body was becoming over stretched physically. It was time to sell up and come home.

Before he came home though there was one more impact on his life that again fuelled, just like with Cambodia, a crusade that was to take him well past legal barriers. During his spells in the USA he had met many of his family of abuse survivors. He had listened first hand to some harrowing tales. He had listened to the hardships caused in their lives many years later, women in their fifties still having functional problems resulting from abuse as a child.

This was now 1996. The internet was expanding at an unbelievable rate and with it the proliferation of child abuse web sites, paedophile rings finding the internet a perfect breeding ground and child portrait photographers finding it a convenient marketing space to meet some of their less desirable customers. Even in America law enforcement was slow to catch on, in Britain it was almost non-existent. This angered his friends so bitterly, almost as if their pain was again being ignored as it was so often when they were children. Within David it hit all his compassionate nerve endings. It was to fuel an obsession that eclipsed everything that had gone on before and was to lead to the most devastating chapter in his life.

Chapter 8:
Charity begins, and ends, at home

Retirement began and ended in 1996. Jo had found a new home, a large Georgian rectory completely in need of refurbishment. In typical manic style he was not interested in a long drawn out loving restoration. In 5 months up to 35 tradesmen restored the building from top to bottom. But still that nagging discontent inside, that feeling of inadequacy, of needing to prove himself.

In March 1997 it was all change again. He was approached by a couple of trustees of a charity that provided counselling and emotional support to abused, limited life and educationally challenged children. This charity was in moribund condition, virtually bankrupt, without a chairman, treasurer and secretary and, as he was to discover later, operating in contravention of its trust deed. This was his chance to do something for his abuse family survivors. He threw himself into restoring this charities fortunes at one time fulfilling all three vacant executive roles, tirelessly drumming up support, restoring it back to financial health, bringing it into line legally, increasing the number of volunteer counsellors and finding and appointing a whole new management team.

The hot topic of the day was a book published by a renowned child photographer called David Hamilton. This book, published in 1995, had been opposed by just about every child welfare organisation as it featured pubescent girls in what many considered to be salacious poses, however the obscene publication squad had deemed it legal art and it was now on open sale in high street bookshops. David opposed this with a passion and used all his contacts in his survivors' family to oppose it in the USA, its biggest market, and in France where David Hamilton now had his home and where his website was based. As the email traffic between himself and friends in the United States increased so many of his family "reciprocated" by sending back to him details of other European websites featuring "artistic" type material and also including websites hosting contents of a less artistic nature including details of a German teenagers website featuring her and her boyfriend. It was all to no avail. There was universal agreement amongst law enforcement across the world that the Hamilton photographs were artistic, not pornographic.

Other charitable involvements followed. 1n 1998 the couple was asked to help a young person who had fallen on hard times and was homeless. He became aware of the miserable cycle of most homeless people. No fixed address = no job, no job = no income, no income = no deposit to put down for a rented home which means no fixed address.

In 1994 the company he helped found had become a public company and the holdings he still held in that company had made the couple moderately wealthy. They had resolved to give one half of their wealth away, One part of that half they shared amongst close family but a large slice was placed into trust to form a charitable foundation that could assist other charities by making small grants or donations. Using funds from this trust he purchased a large house and converted it into 8 small flats, the intention being to rent them off at a nominal rent, waiving the need for deposits, to allow people the chance to get back on their feet.

At the end of 1998 he also used the trust to acquire another property, a large manor house being sold off by a local authority. His charity offering counselling to children facing difficult circumstances was becoming homeless, the owners of the derelict building it was housed in wanting to redevelop. The new home for his charity would be in a delightful parkland setting and the building could undergo redevelopment to provide purpose built facilities making it one of the best facilities of its kind anywhere in the UK.

He not only combined his efforts to the UK. He travelled widely, in Eastern Europe and in Africa he saw the worst ravages that war and totalitarian regimes could inflict on Children, orphans being caged in horrific "hospitals" and orphanages, street children exploited in every conceivable way and he did his utmost to raise awareness back home and in individual countries including raising donations of money and gifts of chocolate and sweets which he personally took to the places where aid was most needed.

A few other charitable involvements followed, he ended up working for the welfare of abused horses and other equines, helping write a lottery application for another charity, helping with business plans of other charities and by the end of 1998 he was again extended to exhaustion point. He still worked with his survivors, often being online to the United States throughout the night.

During this period another unhappy aspect entered David's life. The large house they had moved into had cellars. David had always had a weakness for alcohol. Often an alcoholic haze provided the only mask he could hide his feelings with and even socially he attacked alcohol with the same ferocity as he attacked everything else. His ability to drink most people under the table was legendary, and, of course, enforced the appearance of a macho exterior

David had always quite liked wine and was quite knowledgeable on the subject. Now he decided he would become a wine collector. Not any old wine collector though, he had to be one of the best. The biggest, the most extravagant, the most varied, the most complex and the most knowledgeable, certainly one of them at least.

The wine bins in the cellars were enlarged, capacity for stored bottles rose from 400 to 3,500. In addition there was storage pallets provided for cases holding another 360 bottles. As if he didn't have enough pressure in life he enrolled at a leading London wine and spirits institute and started a series of wine studies, culminating in being awarded a diploma. He became a leading figure at international auction houses such as Sotheby's and Christies. He was regularly invited to wine events and was a familiar figure although unlike others he never sampled a mouthful of wine and then spit it out, his habit of swallowing it and then often going back for more was seen as just a minor eccentricity.

With typical obsessive behaviour the wines would be classified, David's records on what was in his cellar would run into hundreds of pages, analysed by colour, source, vineyard, producer, type of grape, year, price, there was no end of ways he could totally immerse himself into analysing what lay below his feet and then tour the internet looking for supplies of what he felt should be below his feet but was missing from the collection. However it was not what was below his feet that mattered. It was what was brought up from the cellar that was to become an unwelcome and unhealthy influence in his life.

David's occasional foray's into excessive drinking was now to become more than just occasional. With an almost inexhaustible supply of wine below him it was to become a habit bordering on an addiction. It was to become a rarity for an evening to go by without a bottle being opened for dinner and often another bottle being opened as he relaxed in after-dinner conversation with Jo, (relaxed as far as he possibly could. Most times conversations with David was a one way affair of an intense and forceful torrent regarding his latest crusade). Very often if he was working late into the night or online in counselling sessions with one of his survivor family in the United States another bottle of wine would be his companion. Over the next few years alcohol was not only going to seriously affect an already flawed judgement process it was going to affect many other areas of his life including his health.

1999 started as a disaster. Whilst on holiday in the Caribbean they learned that David's father had died. Flying home they tried to contact one of their sons. This son, Adam, the Son who had been their back up on the first of their marathon walks a few years earlier, had been going through a very stressful period. Finding release by spending hours in internet chat rooms he had met a woman over twice his age who lived in America. As the relationship had grown warmer so she had flown to the UK to be with him at the end of 1998. David and Jo were to find out that whilst they were on holiday their son and his friend had flown to Las Vegas, had become married in one of the quickie marriage parlours in that city and were now living near some of her family in California. Jo was devastated.

At the same time this emotional upheaval was taking place so the two housing projects had reached a major stage, two large and complex redevelopments were underway taking practically all his time up. Even though David had been trying to extricate himself from his survivors forum he contacted some of his survivor family members who lived on the West Coast of America to try and help him find his son and report on the conditions he was living in. They were successful. Contact was re-established and

David was ready to attempt reconciliation. That summer, from June to August he criss-crossed the Atlantic over and over again, 3 times in June alone, to visit his son and his wife, an exhausting schedule at the best of times but with everything else going on with his charities it was bringing him physically to breaking point again.

Whilst this was going on David often stayed with members of his forum family in California or Washington State. He learnt that one of their "family" members, the same woman who had complained so vociferously about the website featuring the German teenager in 1997 was experiencing serious emotional and mental health problems. One of the issues she had become obsessively concerned about was the flood of junk mail arriving in her email box day in day out advertising "Child art sites". It was as though her abuse as a child was coming back to haunt her. This planted a seed in his brain that in his exhausted state continued to grow despite the obvious dangers.

Around the end of 1999 the government had at last responded to the clamour to take action against the flood of child pornography and entered into a voluntary agreement with Internet Service Providers to restrict access to a number of newsgroups that blatantly acted as an exchange forum for paedophiles. They did nothing about the "glossy page" websites though that peddled their version of "child art", in many ways jumping on the Hamilton bandwagon of a few years earlier and presumably just as legal. The argument always offered was these websites were located in dubious places outside of first world international law. To David this smacked of just a cheap excuse by bureaucrats to avoid confronting a complex and difficult problem.

At the beginning of 2000 a particular newsgroup caught his attention, one not on the government proscribed list. Newsgroups can be likened to those message boards on public display in places like supermarkets. Anyone can post whatever they like on there, anyone can read whatever they like, they are freely available in the public domain, do not require membership, do not require payment and do not require any details of viewer or poster. As the boards get full so the older messages are removed to make way for new ones being posted on.

This newsgroup had in it over 17,000 images. Up to 2,000 new images were being posted daily. Virtually all of the images were placed there by commercial websites advertising their product. Most of the images were formed into groups of about 150 images, all of a teenage girl dressed in a variety of pseudo-artistic costumes and adopting pseudo-artistic poses. Each group was named after the teenage model and dozens of different websites were involved. As his curiosity deepened he started to notice a pattern, whilst each group of images started with the girl quite innocently dressed, towards the end the uniforms grew scantier until becoming non-existent. He also noticed something else, despite being on different websites under different names the same child models appeared over and over again.

He was intrigued by this and started to note the groups of websites each child appeared in and followed this up by visiting the front page of each website. Hidden away in the small print, underneath the "Members enter here" and "Register here" buttons was the name of the website owner. All tracks led back to a Ukrainian company called studio 13 Art. Using a standard internet search engine he was able to find with complete ease everything anyone needed to know about this company. It was registered in the Ukraine, the names of all the directors were publicly available, its financial records were publicly available, it proclaimed itself to be a co-operative, each of the teenage models receiving a share of the profits paid into a trust fund and it was completely open about the nature of its business. Hitherto the popular conception that was encouraged to exist was that nothing could be done about child-art websites as most of them operated from remote servers hidden away in deserts or jungles of third world countries outside the reach of first world legal jurisdiction yet here was a company operating totally openly in a country that was a candidate member of the European Union, complying apparently with all international legislation and presumably as with Hamilton it was totally legal and untouchable.

His curiosity settled and having more than enough to do elsewhere he moved on. However his curiosity was rekindled at the start of 2002 when he received an email. This email was from someone who it turned out had been on a telephone chat line for people based in northern England, he had had a "special interest" private conversation with someone who had given him an email address which he had either written down incorrectly and sent to David or, more likely, he had been deliberately misled and given the address of someone who it was known would respond appropriately.

At first the contents seemed perfectly innocent if bizarre, this person was apparently organising a party in the Leeds/Halifax area and needed some female company for the party goers, about 9 to 13 girls it appeared. David wrote back saying basically "sorry, wrong person, best of luck" but something about the way the email was phrased intrigued him. Reading it again he wrote back to this person asking if he really meant girls AGED 9 to 13. He received an affirmative reply and immediately contacted West Yorkshire police in Leeds. He copied all correspondence to them and was contacted a few days later and asked if he would help with their inquiries by keeping this person talking, acting as if he could supply what this person wanted and basically extracting what information he could about claims this person had done it before, knew there were people who could arrange such things etc. He did this for three weeks, typically with complete disregard to his own security, at the end of which West Yorkshire police advised him their background investigations were completed, a file was being passed on to the National Criminal Investigation Service, thank you for your help and "we are sure NCIS will be in touch shortly to offer their thanks as well".

They did eventually get in touch, but not to offer their thanks.

By 2002 even David knew he had become over-committed and was driving himself into another physical collapse. He started to reduce his many charitable commitments but that raging discontent inside needed an outlet. He decided to agitate to move home, his arguments being if he was going to retire then why not do it in a country with a warmer climate and a less onerous taxation burden.

Jo was heartbroken at the thought of moving home. She had put her heart and soul into their house, it was where her roots were, but there was something attractive about a fresh start and one final challenge before old age took over. They debated where in the world to look, the United States had always held an attraction for them both, David knew of a lovely little town in Virginia, last resting places of two of the most renowned military commanders of the civil war. They found a house there and made plans to move.

In August that year the couple heard some devastating news. Their Son Adam, a gifted microlight aircraft pilot, had taken someone on a check flight around the local airfield near Sacramento, California. This person had panicked whilst at the controls but had refused to allow Adam to regain control and in the resulting crash Adam had been severely injured, his right hand almost being severed, his left hand sliced in two and multiple fingers severed. He had been airlifted to a leading centre of reconstructive surgery in San Francisco where repairs to his hands were carried out in an 11 hour operation. Jo and David flew out on the first available flight to San Francisco and throughout August and

September shuttled backwards and forwards as their son struggled to get back to health.

Throughout the last part of the year they also shuttled backwards and forwards between the USA and the UK preparing their house, moving some of their home furnishings and artefacts over, and at the beginning of the following year were fast becoming resident. They were in Virginia on the 9th of January when David took a phone call from his secretary. "Are you somewhere private?" she asked. "Yes" he replied, "why?". "I have bad news" she replied, "The police have raided your home".

David and Jo flew back on the first available flight. He was blissfully unaware of the holocaust he was flying home to and together with Jo had decided that whatever the accusations they would rely on legal aid. They both knew of his innocence and had a belief in the infallibility of United Kingdom justice and both felt that the one thing that must be seen is that wealth does not buy freedom, innocence does.

The following Tuesday with his legal aid Lawyer David attended the local police station for interview. It lasted for a couple of hours, consisted mostly of acknowledging that the computers and other peripherals that had been seized belonged to him and he even nobly volunteered that he took complete responsibility for anything found on them, another mistake that was to blow up in his face and also possibly the only inaccurate thing he offered for almost anyone could freely access his computers when visiting either his main home or his London flat. At the end of the interview he was told the investigation was caused by his credit card being used for a number of transactions with a website based in the United States called landslide, these transactions taking place in June 1999.

He had never heard of landslide, he had never ever paid to go on such a website and June 1999 was the month he was shuttling backwards and forwards to the United States to achieve reconciliation with his Son, of all times not the time he was likely to be sat at home surfing dubious websites. He walked out of the police station confident of the imminent collapse of the investigation.

The police would find no evidence of any material having been downloaded from this website. Years later this national investigation, carried out on a vast scale, would be seen to be seriously flawed by substantial amounts of fraudulent transactions contaminating the evidence. David's own credit card company would later that year confirm that indeed in 1999 a number of internet transactions on his account had been investigated and subsequently found to be fraudulent. A few years later a Cambridge Professor and security expert would pose the question regarding this nationwide investigation of "was this the worst UK policing scandal ever?" It would all be too late for David. His nightmare was about to get worse, much worse. All those compassionate activities of the past that just a few days ago would have been widely applauded were to come to haunt him.

Finding no evidence of what they came looking for, the police attention became focussed on other material found on his computers, material accumulated from all those activities of the past. It now mattered little that he had been a leading campaigner to have the Hamilton books banned, evidence was found that he had once had Hamilton images on his computer and even though these images were still considered legal when published in a book, a book to this day still on open sale on the high street, they were to be deemed illegal when recorded onto computer media belonging to him.

Equally, Studio 13 material, still at that time on open access in the UK, sold openly through a number of websites operated from another European Country and without condemnation, censure or "public heath warnings" from the

UK or any other European country, were now to be deemed to be illegal.

Much of the allegations would have been ludicrously funny had it not been so serious. Amongst the allegations were images allegedly made on his home desktop computer that on the evidence of stamps in his passport alone it could be proved he could not possibly of made, those stamps showing entry into countries often thousands of miles from home. Some of these allegations even included images made when he was not only 2,500 miles away on board the QE2 cruising around the Caribbean but also at that exact date and time so merry from the party on board he could not even be capable of switching a computer on let alone do anything with it!

The local media did not help, his name constantly being linked to reporting of the odious material described in lurid detail as being available from the website that was the subject of the original investigation and at no time was it ever made public no material from that website had been found or indeed any evidence discovered that he had ever gone there.

Soon malicious rumour and gossip, much of it coming directly from police sources, disclosing private and unrelated correspondence found on his computers, began to sweep through the small community where they lived. The most sensitive and private information of the sort that many have on their computers, information totally unrelated to the investigation, was being made available as a source of public gossip.

They were fortunate. Friends, neighbours and family showed unflinching support and as that year dragged on so that support grew stronger and more protective, many urging David to do for himself just as he had done so often for others and stand up to injustice. However the constant media spotlight, the constant barrage of grossly inaccurate reporting, the constant circulation of rumour and innuendo was to take its toll and it was not only David who suffered, for months he was to watch Jo's health and mental well-being deteriorate. The effects on him watching this was just too much.

After 9 months of the most vindictive and intense mental pressure he had reached the end. He was almost broken mentally and had reached a stage of physical exhaustion where rational decision making was almost impossible. Jo was on the verge of physical and mental breakdown and his concern for her health was becoming a constant worry to him. Vigilante action fuelled by that grossly inaccurate reporting and fanned by that malicious gossip was a distinct possibility. The only way he could fight on was to move out of the area to his London flat but that would leave Jo alone and unprotected. He was prepared to take any action, no matter how unjust, to lift the media spotlight to allow him and Jo to just have a normal life.

As his physical and mental well being began to crumble so the walls that had been my prison also started to crumble. As that year approached its close he felt his life was also approaching a closure or at least his life as he had known it. In truth his life had started to end. My life had started to begin.

Chapter 9:
Emergence

THAT awful year was drawing to a close. There had been lots of heart to heart discussions between David and Jo. He promised her faithfully that never ever again would he get so deeply involved in anything that would cause him to lose sight of what danger he could be walking into. He was retired, again, his crusading boots well and truly hung up and this time it was for real.

It was for real. For the first time in his adult life David was going to allow himself to do nothing, allow his brain time to think, allow his mind time to reflect. He was in his flat in London, a flat awaiting refurbishment and living accommodation was Spartan. His bruised exhausted mind was reflecting, not only on that year but on an adult lifetime that was a chronicle of wounds caused by a total inability to see some form of over commitment he was driving into. He was sat on his bed staring into a full length mirror asking over and over again the question "why had his life, so successful and full of joy in so many ways, been such a chronicle of deep unhappiness and a restless churning constantly driving him into danger?" The image in that mirror stared back at him, the mind at last being able to speak, the reply was simple and it was that he was the wrong way round.

It was like a bolt of lightning. Suddenly it was all so obvious. As if all of his adult life had disappeared he was now in a continuum with that child of so many years ago. He was different, not what it said on the packet, he was fighting himself and what he and society perceived him to be.

Over the next few weeks the desire to see himself in female form grew to be overwhelming. At first it was a transvestite escort he visited for a makeover but something wrong with the look, it was not naturally female. He then found a dressing agency specialising in producing the "natural look". He stared into the mirror as the make-up was being applied, half feeling like coco the clown, half feeling very embarrassed. The make up finished he was asked to close his eyes as the hair was put in place. He could feel it being fitted, combed into shape, and then asked to open his eyes. The effect was electrifying. Staring back at him in the mirror was the person he always knew he was. He was looking at me.

During the makeover he had been asked to choose a femme name. They were going through the possibilities. He was recalling those childhood dreams of waking up as a girl and the name of that girl, the girl that was always happy, the girl called Jennifer, the name that seemed to signify happiness. The hair interrupted his chain of thought and he begged to know where he could acquire the same hair. The proprietor came back with the box it had been packed in. Looking at the label she announced that the manufacturer was Rene of Paris and the style was called "Jennifer". Jennifer had met Jennifer. My name for the rest of my life had been chosen.

He returned to his flat, his mind in turmoil. Clearly when he had looked at that reflection in the mirror something had happened inside him, but he was a bloke, why on earth did he want to see himself as a woman? This was just a sleazy unnatural bit of escapism related to wanting to escape all those events of the previous year.

The sleazy unnatural bit of escapism would not go away. The genie was out of the bottle. The feelings inside grew and grew. He started to acquire a wardrobe. He joined an internet fetish chat room as "TV Jenny" but felt so uncomfortable with the transvestite designation he changed his identity and the shortened form of his name calling himself Jenni. This was all being done in secret, without Jo or any of his friends knowing, the feelings of deceit were compounding the anguish inside but as he sank into an identity crisis so the ability to relate to others, even someone as close to him as Jo, started to diminish. He was suffering also massive confusion inside so how could he relate something he could not understand himself?

He needed somewhere to keep Jenni's wardrobe, a friend offered him a short term lease on a small, one bedroomed basement flat near his London home. As much as he felt ashamed and revolted at his behaviour and the world of deceit he was entering into the need to embrace the female persona now known as Jenni grew and grew. Friends from his online chat room came over for dinner, the first time he had ever met anyone else as Jenni with the exception of the people who had first helped him to see her.

A month later those same friends took him as Jenni to a fetish fair. That evening returning home they stopped for dinner just around the corner to the tiny basement flat. This was the first time he as Jenni had been out in a perfectly normal mainstream social environment. As his nerves settled, as he realised that everyone else in the restaurant were just continuing as normal and not staring in shock, disgust or amusement at him something happened. He felt content. Gone was that internal churning agitation that had been part of him for the whole of his life. Gone was that feeling of inadequacy, of being different, of being not quite in step with everyone else. Even though he knew that to most people, including himself, he looked a freak, a joke, a bloke in a frock, despite all those things he, for the first time in his whole life, felt normal.

The pressure within to be living as a female was inexorable but so to was the anguish it was causing. He was a man but when he presented as one his life was one of churning turmoil. When he presented as a female there was a peace and calm inside, but also there was self-disgust at indulging in a sleazy unnatural activity and self-disgust at the growing deceit. It was coming up to nearly a year since Jenni had first manifested herself in him. She was now taking over his life. He had to stop it. He did.

Over the next six months the anguish was unbearable. He could no longer survive just living as a man but he could not return to that sleazy life of living as a female, living in a world of secrecy and deceit. His relationship with Jo was falling apart as the internal churning agitation would make him volatile and unpredictable. The slightest disagreement with her would see him storming off back to their London home leaving Jo becoming more and more certain he was sharing his life with another woman.

Just as it was as a child he could no longer associate with society and being with large groups of people would cause him to become almost hysterical and seek solitude elsewhere. At a meal with most of Jo's family present he had upset everyone by abruptly getting up and leaving the restaurant as the need to be alone, to find isolation, overwhelmed him. Enjoying a short break with Jo caravanning in the Shropshire countryside he had repeatedly stormed off late at night to spend hours sitting somewhere in the middle of nowhere isolated and alone with his thoughts and the screaming pain and anguish inside.

He experienced wave after wave of compulsion to destroy himself, On one occasion he found himself at Hammersmith underground station, his toes literally over the platform edge, his body rocking, his eyes transfixed, staring at those rails, at that live rail that was just half a second away from releasing him into the blackness of death, releasing him from the pain and anguish that was tearing him apart inside. Only a supreme act of will, which he felt to be spiritual, pulled him away from that edge, propelled him towards the exit, led him to safety and a long walk home in pouring rain. He knew that mentally he was falling apart. He knew he had to seek help and obtained a referral to a renowned London clinic specialising in treating mental and psychological illnesses. Ironically it was the same clinic that had cared for him when he was a child.

The doctors he saw recognised a mental state close to breakdown and urged him to accept admittance into a place of safety for him. This he could not do, his secret world would be exposed. The specialists in the first instance diagnosed a form of Post Traumatic Stress disorder, an accumulation of stresses going as far back as to that sudden and traumatic health breakdown that caused early retirement. As they started to chart his life history a pattern of very contrasting peaks and troughs began to emerge. They listened as he described how he always felt the need to run through life at 120 miles an hour and asked was he really running from something at 120 miles an hour.

Internal agitation that causes this sort of behaviour is often caused by repressed sexual problems so they examined him deeply for any form of behaviour associated with repressed sexual orientation. They concluded all was normal and healthy. He had explored, he had experimented but sexually he was comfortable with the heterosexual state he was living in.

The other causes are often gender identity related issues. During this period he had brought Jenni back out of her box. His mind could no longer bear not having the release of peace and calm he felt when he was presenting as female. It was time to overcome the shame and self-loathing and explain about this sleazy desire he had to be female to the psychiatrists and how he felt no longer able to exist in society presenting as a male. It was to them as though someone had turned the lights on.

They started to rebuild his childhood. Bit by bit working on known instances and dates they saw the same pattern emerge that was now apparent in the adult they were treating. Childhood gender dysphoria was indicated in almost every incident. They explained to David that in their opinion he was suffering with gender dysphoria. They went on to explain it would be unlikely he could ever return to living as a male, indeed the likely results would be the misery he was experiencing now would just deepen to where self-destruction or mental breakdown would be inevitable and in the case of the latter it may take many years of in-patient treatment for him to recover and he may also be treated as she rather than he anyway.

It was explained to him that the severity of the gender dysphoria he was suffering with meant it was likely the only way he would be able to live a happy and otherwise normal life in the future was to live in his psychological gender and making whatever physical adjustments were necessary to allow body to be congruent with mind.

They concluded that now it was essential that as a matter of extreme urgency he accepts a referral to either an NHS Gender Identity Clinic or one of the private specialists approved as being competent to diagnose and treat Gender Dysphoria. They emphasised their grave concerns over his mental health and his personal safety and also pointed out they had a duty of care towards him that may cause them to seek other means to ensure his safety, a nice way of saying he could be sectioned into a mental hospital.

He finally agreed he would see at the earliest possibility a Gender specialist and until then he would remain under their close care. He never made that appointment and neither did he go back.

Denial had set in again, a denial made easier now that he had brought Jenni out of her box for now at least he had days when he could again get respite from that raging anguish and enjoy the peace and calm that his life was when as Jenni. He now convinced himself they were wrong, it was not as serious as suggested, its was only a fantasy that had to run its course and if he needed help to wean himself away from the fantasy he would do it in his own time at his own pace when he was ready not when others would dictate.

The denial lasted for a few more weeks then in almost identical circumstances to the previous year he found himself at the same fetish fair before being part of a group returning to that same restaurant near his basement flat. Just as it was the previous year he was hit with that wave of feeling completely, totally normal, of being whole, of being functional rather than dysfunctional.

A couple of days later he had to return to Jo and his main home. This time that feeling of being normal was not something that could be put away. The weight of depression, sadness, dislocation inside was dreadful as he changed back into David. Arriving home he was told a church group meeting was restarting that evening. The thought of people around him was too much. The cry for solitude as he fought his internal pain was too loud, leaving poor Jo again confused, hurt and angry he stormed out of the house and returned to London.

He returned to his little basement flat, Jenni's secret home. Curled up on the settee he agonised over his predicament. He now knew all those specialists were right. This was not a piece of escapism that would disappear as his exhausted mind recovered, this was real, he had a serious gender problem, he needed help but how could he ever disclose his secret sleazy world to anyone, especially the woman he loved, the woman he had been so deceitful to, the woman who would now have to be told that the man she had lived with for over 30 years was really a female? Yet there was no way back, the thought of continuing to live as that anguished male was just too awful to contemplate. As day turned into night he could see no way out. The isolation was screamingly painful. There was no one he could talk to or release to. He had no life worth living for, either alternative being unacceptable according to his confused and exhausted mind. He needed to talk to someone.

He dialled a number and poured his heart out to the person at the other end. She was a volunteer with the organisation known as the Samaritans. She could only listen, no advice, no being told what to do, just listen and he cried and talked and cried again. Finally exhausted he put the phone down and fell asleep. The following day it did not seem quite so bleak, he knew he had to talk to Jo. He knew he needed the specialist help he was so exhorted to seek a few weeks ago.

He now knew what he had to do. First his mind needed help, to understand the savage conflicts going on inside, to reconcile the him in his life with the her who refused to go away. He contacted a psychotherapist who specialised in gender problems and made an appointment for the earliest possible time. He now needed to tell Jo and again the obstacles to finding the opportunity, to present this whole passage of pain and deceit in the right way, seemed overwhelming. The respite was short lived. He started to slide back into that dark place where he felt there was no way forward, no way back, no life worth living.

Both Jo and he, after this latest turbulent bout, had reached the conclusion that their marriage in this current set of circumstances was unviable. In the solitude of his basement flat he started to think of the unthinkable, a future without Jo. This only plunged him into a greater and deeper spiral of despair. One evening He made arrangements to meet a friend for dinner, someone who like him had experienced Post Traumatic Stress Disorder, a friend he could explain his feelings to and at the same time listen to this friend recount hers. It was mutual support for each other.

The night before he had plunged into another deep bout of despair and isolation but the following morning had managed to shake off the feelings of disturbance this would normally produce. He got through the day and enjoyed an evening in the company of his friend. The mutual support had worked and he was feeling a bit stronger. Returning to his basement flat he was aware he had been without his mobile phone and had not been able to ring Jo, something he did every evening normally without fail, there might have been unendurable tension amongst them at this time but they both still felt that need to talk to each other.

He switched on his mobile and saw the "messages waiting" alert. The first was a message from Jo asking what the hell was that message left on his mobile answering service all about? The next was from Nanette, his secretary, pleading to know where he was. The next was from Jo again, basically David, please get in touch. The next was from Nanette saying she was with Jo driving to London, please get in touch. The last two were strident pleas from Jo saying she was at their London flat, please; please get in touch, then a WPC from the local police station asking him to please get in touch with the police.

His mind whirled. The calls all related to something left as the answer phone greeting on his mobile but whilst events of the night before were a memory of deep distress and despair the specifics of those memories were vague and hazy, specifics having been wiped out by a brain that really did not want to go there. He tried to access his greeting, his hands were shaking, his mind barely functioning and in his almost panicky rush to listen to his message he deleted it. He was never to hear what had been left.

He dialled Jo's mobile. A deeply distressed Jo almost screamed at him to come home, then explained the content of his message he had left as a greeting. It was a two minute mono-syllabic drone basically saying goodbye to those he loved. Jo had heard it, confided in the local parish priest who shared her view it was deeply distressing and definitely not just a cry for help, it conveyed real intent. Jo had then turned to Nanette, David's secretary, someone who probably outside of his immediate family knew the workings of his mind more than anyone. Nan concurred with the priest, this was not the David she knew, this was gravely serious, together she and Jo had set off straight away to come and find him. Arriving at their London flat they found no trace of David there, not surprising as David had spent the last two nights in Jenni's secret basement flat. In desperation they had contacted the police who on hearing the answering message concurred this was serious and had immediately posted David as an at risk missing person.

David then spoke to one of the two police women who had first interviewed Jo. They asked where he was and could he meet them at the local police station. David agreed but insisted they met outside first; going into police stations brought back some rather bad memories for him.

The policewomen turned up and persuaded him to go inside to an interview room. It was obvious to them both that sat in front of them was someone who was seriously ill, who was seriously at risk from himself. They exhorted David to allow them to take him to a place of safety, a hospital where he could be cared for. He screamed inside to say yes, nothing he wanted more than to be released from this unendurable pain he found himself struggling with, but then the secret would be out, the decision he couldn't face making would be made for him, no, he had to say no, had to ask to be returned to Jo and his secretary. It was not that easy. The police had a duty of care, their first responsibility was for David to be safe even if this meant having him admitted to a place of safety for his own protection against his own will. For two hours they exhorted him to go with them, to agree to voluntary admittance, for two hours he inwardly screamed to say yes but outwardly felt he had to refuse, they talked to Jo and Nanette, talked to the hospital, weighed up all the pro's and cons and finally agreed to release him into Jo and Nanette's custody.

Reunited with Jo and Nanette they returned home the following morning. He still did not feel able to confide in Jo, still was not ready but the door had been opened for that opportunity to take place, the end of the whole nightmare had begun. Jo now knew that there was a terrible conflict inside him. David knew it was only a matter of time before the source of that conflict would be divulged.

The opportunity came from an unexpected source. Jo's Mum, at the age of 81, decided she was going to see Australia, to go to the wedding of her grand-niece and to stop with a niece she had not seen for many years. Whilst stopping with her niece she learned of a family secret. Jo's Uncle, her Mum's brother, had been a closet transvestite for most of his life. On her return back to England she confided in Jo who immediately sprung to her uncles defence, basically "what harm has it done, who has he hurt, if it brings him happiness then good for him and just whose business is it anyway?

Hearing Jo's defence of her uncle was to David like hearing Jo turn a key in a lock. Time and time again in after dinner discussions he would return to the subject of Jo's uncle and family reaction. Finally one evening the conversation took the right course. He was unusually relaxed that evening, Jo had felt more relaxed and more willing to step on thorny ground. She asked an innocent question anticipating a sharp retort from the most non-effeminate, macho man she knew. "Have you ever thought or been tempted to cross-dress" she asked, smiling. The response was not what she expected.

He told her the whole story, what gender dysphoria was, how he now had an appointment to see a gender specialist, how his only hope for a normal life was to transition from being male to being female. Jo had no reservations despite the awful consequences for her. She saw her life was with the person she had married. She wanted him well even if that meant he was now her. She embraced the new person in her life. With that embrace I was at last able to escape from my prison. I had been released.

Chapter 10:
No longer David, not quite Jenni

IT was to be a few months before I started the process of transitioning properly. Firstly Jo and I had to get to know each other. Our first meeting was in a restaurant near my secret flat in London, a restrained difficult affair, She wondering who the hell was the dreadfully dressed and dreadfully made up caricature sat in front of her and me holding back desperate feelings of shame and embarrassment.

I don't know what went wrong that night. We had travelled to London together and had stayed together at our London flat but then I had taken myself off to Jenni's basement to get myself ready for the evening. I was dreadfully nervous, this the first time Jo was to meet Jenni. Everything I had meant to wear, mostly the most demure clothes in my wardrobe, somehow seemed out of place. I ended up putting on a most awful bright red skirt, something bought for 99 pence on eBay, something that finished well above my knees, shiny stockings, a black tarty top that wouldn't quite button up properly showing off liberal amounts of my male beer belly and all worn underneath a wig that resembled something belonging to a mid-1960's teenager. I looked dreadful.

Either way the following day Jo and Jen went on their first shopping trip together, an incredible act of courage by Jo who must have been acutely embarrassed being seen with this caricature. She must of also have been quite fearful of the reaction it was likely to attract. I returned home with a sensible dark brown skirt from Marks and Spencer's and some bits to make my hair look something more suitable for someone obviously over the age of 16.

I was still holding on to my masculinity, after all I had spent the last 40 years of my life proving to everyone including myself that I was a bloke, a macho bloke, a mans man. A lifetime of conditioning and nurturing does not disappear just because a Doctor says "you are female, now go and act and live like one". I still refused to believe it was all true and I was still partially in denial. Still hoping that it was all a bit of escapism and I might wake up one morning and could be David again.

I was continuing to see the psychotherapist I had turned to at the end of that dreadful period of emergence, the person who more than anyone kept me sane through that period and was to be my rock through transition. He had meticulously broken down the conflicting walls inside, David who loathed Jenni and Jenni who wanted rid of her jailor, to finally rebuild both as one person, a person beginning to feel strong again, being able to emerge from that desperately dark tunnel I had been in. Bit by bit the walls came down, we actually discovered that in many of his responses David was quite transphobic which explains the difficulties he had when I started to break free of my prison.

Jo meanwhile had been on a number of internet help lines for nearest and dearest of people facing transition. What she read and saw was a catalogue after catalogue of wrecked and broken marriages, tale after tale of sexual orientation changing once that femininity is released or hormone therapy started. It was a desperately anxious time for her and my often irrational behaviour did nothing to help.

It was to take four more miserable months and three more specialists before I could finally accept it myself and it was to be a most difficult four months for our relationship.

There is a belief held by many people working in gender medicine, psychotherapists, psychiatrists, psychologists and other psych's that regardless of the chronological age of the individual the person that emerges during the transitional period starts off at the development age of a pubescent child and indeed a lot of the interviews I had in all the roads to diagnosis had often centred around establishing whether I had any particular fascination with the behaviour patterns associated with young teenagers. For Poor Jo this certainly appeared to be the case. This poor woman, whose life had been made a misery before, now had a flouncing teenaged drama queen half wanting to be a bloke and half wanting to be a woman living with her. The clothes were wrong, the hair was wrong, the way I walked was wrong, the language I used was wrong but each time Jo tried to point something out I would storm off in a tantrum. The stresses upon us in this "pre-transition" period were enormous.

During this period we had chosen to tell a few friends and family. The story of life of many people going through transition is one of rejection and heartbreak, close friends and family not understanding the causes of Gender Dysphoria, not understanding the medical basis and living with the myth it is a lifestyle choice somehow related to sexuality. The reaction so often is to disassociate with people considered freaks by a large part of a sometimes bigoted and ignorant society. Jo and I realised this was the most important part of transition, it could not be hurried, would involve sacrifice, would often involve spending day after day, weekend after weekend, laboriously explaining all those issues and medical causes most people would be totally ignorant about, as I once was. We also felt that people who had stood by us in moments of great adversity deserved the respect of being told in person, not hearing it on the grapevine, not having it suddenly shoved in their faces.

It was to be a laborious, often frustrating, business. A typical routine would be Saturday night, Dinner with David and Jo, a two hour pre-dinner discussion on Gender Dysphoria, dinner, more discussion, the same questions answered over and over again with as much integrity and respect for the questioner as possible, then often meeting again the following day, the poor stunned visitors having had time to digest the incredible news, returning for lunch, afternoon tea, or dinner only this time with Jo and Jenni.

We were to be blessed beyond measure. Couple after couple blinked in shock when they first heard, listened attentively to the causes and effects of Gender Dysphoria, showed concern for above all Jo who had been through so much and now in many ways was going to have to take the brunt of all of this and finally offered full unconditional support. Slowly my mind began to adjust that this was for real, it could succeed and there was light at the end of the tunnel. Gradually I started to inch towards that final acceptance in my own mind that would allow me to make that decision to accept transition as the way forward.

As my confidence grew and the support of those dearest to us began to mount we could at last address some fundamental issues of our own. Jo needed to know just where it would all end and whilst I could say that Gender Reassignment surgery was still only a distant consideration we both knew that it could be eventually unavoidable. Up to this point I still was in partial denial and I was still believing myself and convincing others that transition could be a partial objective, as long as I could spend some time as Jenni I would still be able to live as some of the time as David. Jo was more level headed and fully understood that from now on she would have to look to sharing a life with someone who had a female body.

I also needed constant reassurance that the pain I was causing Jo really was necessary; there was no way to fully return to gender. However it was becoming increasingly necessary for both of us that I started to move on. I was living a life of limbo, sometimes David, sometimes Jenni. It was living two lives. In my London home when arriving dressed as David it had to be furtive and secretive to avoid those who only knew Jenni, in our main home it was having to arrive as David so as to keep my transition a secret until those important to us had been told.

On one visit to the South Coast town where my family lives I changed six times. I left our home as David, arriving at our flat in London changed into Jenni, drove to Brighton, checked into the hotel, changed into David to visit my sister who at that time could not accept Jenni, returned to the hotel to get changed so I could meet with a friend who only ever knew me as Jenni before changing into David so I could visit my Mum, then very ill and unable to be told. Returning exhausted and confused to the hotel late that evening I felt I needed a drink before finally going to bed so I changed into Jenni for a late-night drink in the bar. I was not only going through an identity crisis Max Factor was going through a supply crisis trying to keep me stocked up with make-up.

Jo was seeing a Consultant psychotherapist at a Gender Identity Clinic nearby. He had offered Jo emotional support and as he was also an ordained priest he was someone Jo felt she could comfortably confide in. He listened to Jo describe a terrible story of her life in recent years and professed huge admiration for her courage and fortitude in the face of a catalogue of disasters and relationship difficulties that would of broken many. He finally over the next few weeks reached a point where felt he needed to talk to me if he was to be able to help Jo further.

He, with Jo's permission, agreed to talk to me, something I welcomed for this would be the first time that Jo and I would be able to bare our souls collectively to someone who was not only a highly respected consultant but someone who also possessed huge humanitarian values and beliefs. He listened to my history, a synopsis of all that had gone on before, agreed with everyone else, yes it was Gender Dysphoria, it was primary meaning I was born with the condition and symptoms were there as a child before the onset of puberty, He also recognised that I had an intense need now to just move on, step forward from the denial, accept who and what I was and begin the process of rebuilding my life, our lives, on a solid foundation and not on the shifting sands of trying to be something I wasn't or worse attempting a compromise between the two people that I had become and until recently had been at war with each other.

By sharing with this incredible man my innermost fears in front of Jo I could see more clearer than ever that I just had to come off the fence, the need to live as one person was paramount, the need to just be Jenni was paramount. The need to accept whatever diagnosis was made and stick to that decision with focussed discipline was paramount.

I had to come off the fence. More and more the times I was retreating back to being David was causing great internal anguish resulting in bouts of petulant tantrum that was beginning to wear down Jo. This consultant agreed and made the necessary arrangements to send me for one more referral, to one of the most eminent private psychiatrists in the country.

The day arrived. It was just over 4 months since I had first told Jo about my feminine persona. I was sat with this specialist who spoke with great calm authority, who knew, had seen many times before people with the same stresses as me. He had for a couple of hours interviewed me and referred to the very copious historical notes that travelled with me. He concluded there was no doubt whatsoever I had Gender Dysphoria and it was a primary condition. All my previous assertions that it was only fantasy, a need to escape from those awful events a couple of years earlier and the only help I needed was to be guided back to normality were debunked by this specialist who had pointed out all the evidence from childhood onwards of gender dysphoria that had been apparent long before the police investigation that had driven David to the edge and allowed my prison walls to come tumbling down.

He now turned to my current situation of trying to live in limbo.

He asked was it fair on Jo to keep this limbo going. She had been devastated by my erratic behaviour during the period of emergence, further devastated by hearing I was Gender Dysphoric and would have to undergo changes; the least she deserved now was a stable platform to move forward on. For myself, how long did I want to keep beating myself up? The very happiness and contentment I feel when presenting myself in my true psychological identity of female surely says everything when compared to that anguished frantic male rushing around at 120 miles an hour. In summary his words were "You are now Jennifer, there is no way back, yes its tough, life is tough, deal with it".

His words hit home. I accepted his diagnosis. I accepted I would start the process of medically supervised transition under his care and direction. There would be now no turning back.

Chapter 11
Transition

There is a belief with many people that people like me, whether male to female or female to male, transition because we choose to, that it's all a matter of choice. Nothing can be further from the truth. I would do anything to avoid transition, if I could have taken a gender pill that would have allowed me to continue living happily as a male I would have walked barefoot for a thousand miles on broken glass to get it. I know of no one who would choose to transition if there was an acceptable alternative. I, and others like me, transition because there is no other alternative left if we are to have a life, or indeed continue living for the biggest cause of premature death amongst people like me is suicide.

Transition is hell. It's a time when you find out who really are your friends, who's still going to be there at the end. It's the time of knowing what family love and loyalty is, or is not. It's a time of physical pain and mental turmoil, of self-questioning and self-doubt. It's a time when the full brunt of ignorance, bigotry and prejudice will hit right in the face. A time when just going out to do the normal everyday things will be a time of apprehension, of not knowing if this is going to be the day to be sneered or jeered at, backs turned, spat at, verbally assaulted, physically threatened or become a victim of a hate crime.

I was to be fortunate. Transition for me was to be relatively easy and at the end all my family would still be there, all but a couple of my original friends would still be there and Jo and I would make many more friends along the way. Sadly for many though it's a time of heartbreak, fear, pain and defeat, a defeat that often ends in suicide.

There is a thing called the Real Life Test. A requirement for anyone going through transition is to spend a minimum of 12 months, 24 months if being treated by the NHS, living full time in the new gender role before any irreversible treatment can take place. This is to ensure that once changes start to become permanent the person undergoing those changes is completely comfortable with living in the assigned gender.

It can be quite a brutal process. Even though we still had a lot of close friends and family to talk to and it was going to be a few months yet before David could be put away forever the process really started after that final confirming consultation. Prior to this moment my life as Jenni had been in the safe confines of either of my homes, out in public with a large group of friends or the very occasional solo walk down the busy high road in London where my flat is and where I had become a reasonably well known figure, not that it mattered, in a city so cosmopolitan as London I could walk down that high road or any other high road with three heads and begging for change so I could ring home and no one would of noticed.

My first test would be what forever more I would christen the Tesco test, although it was in fact Sainsbury's, either way I needed some mundane every day groceries. No longer could I just wipe the make up off, get changed into David and toddle off to my local supermarket. From now on it was only as Jenni.

I was hardly equipped for my first close-quarter solo foray into everyday mainstream society. I walked like someone labouring under a 60kg rucksack, hardly elegant at the best of times in the high mountain passes but tripping down the high road in a skirt and heels most definitely not the image one would wish to cultivate. I had a very dark beard shadow, the only make up I could use to cover it up was something akin to theatrical greasepaint, the gloss taken off with liberal applications of powder put on with something resembling a decorators paint brush, large size. Various shades of blushers would adorn this blanked canvas, the need to disguise the beard shadow ruling out at this stage what would become my mantra regarding make-up later on that less is more. My choice of lipstick normally revolved around one of a number of shades of bright red, often clashing hideously with my choice of eye shadow which normally created the exquisite impression of someone who had gone six rounds in a boxing ring with someone rather large and rather heavy.

The clothes did not give me much hope of going unnoticed either. My development age had come on in leaps and bounds, I had progressed from pubescent teenager to an early twenties flouncing tart in weeks but it did mean the skirt hemline finished somewhere between chest and kneecaps. The chest itself was a sight for sore eyes. Like most people in my position I had to wear a bra padded out with various bits of silicone and foam accessories, often called chicken fillets, although in my case the chicken fillets resembled sides of beef in terms of elegant proportions.

Finishing it all off my voice was most definitely male. However the Real Life Test is just that, it is a test of living in real life not in a fantasy bubble, it takes no prisoners, if you are going to do it then get on and do it.

After an hour settling my nerves it was time for this picture of feminine allure to step out of the front door and to launch Jenni onto an unsuspecting public. As feared I was easily read, the checkout operator fumbling with the schools voucher practically giving me the whole book, but nothing untoward, no hostility, no jeers, no laughter, just mild curiosity. It was an overwhelming experience. Here I was doing something just so mundane and ordinary it would be laughable but the feeling that swept over me I can only describe as liberation. I just felt so free, as though a huge weight had come off my shoulders, Again, even knowing people were looking at me with "what in heavens name is that" type stares I felt totally, completely normal.

I didn't want to go home but then why should I? David would have been programmed, three and a quarter minutes walk there, 8 minutes shopping, 3 minutes checkout (and if it was more than four minutes then basket dumped on the floor and walking out empty handed mumbling something about "I don't do queuing") three and a quarter minutes back, seventeen and a half minutes in total, a precious seventeen and a half minutes he could have been totally immersed in his latest project.

Not so with Jenni, I was a liberated female now, sorry, now I'm out its going to be a saunter down the high street window shopping. It did not matter what I had to be home for, I just wanted more and more and more of this intoxicating feeling of being liberated, free, normal and complete, myself at long last.

In times to come I would meet bigotry and prejudice, be verbally abused, be chased down the street with someone running behind me shouting "You ***ing tranny, you should be locked away". In one week on an internet site I was abused relentlessly culminating in a death threat that even the forum operators felt necessary to report to the police. I have to say though the vast majority of the British public quite justifiably deserve their reputation for fair-minded tolerance.

I also started facial depilation, a process to remove my beard. There are two main techniques, Electrolysis where a fine needle is inserted into the hair follicle and a high voltage charge sent down it cauterising the blood vessels that nourish the follicle, or absorbed light technology, either Laser or Intense Pulsed light techniques, where intense light is absorbed by the hair follicle which is then basically burnt away. This is a quicker technique than electrolysis but does not work on grey hair and sadly I had a lot of them. However I had a need to get things done quickly and as light source depilation is much quicker than electrolysis so I opted for that despite the grey hair. Whichever procedure is opted for there is one truth for both, it hurts, and even using the quicker technique it was going to be 15 months of pain before my beard finally went during which at one time putting lipstick on was agony for two weeks after having half my lip burnt and blistered by the laser.

Another intense source of pain at the beginning was my feet. They are big, even for a bloke, and they are wide. Delicate narrow fitting ladies fashions even with a modest low heel put me through agonies until by trial and error I found those styles and those retailers where I could walk more than a couple of hundred yards in comfort. It sounds laughable, and often was, but for many months walking anywhere was an act of painful endurance.

I was placed on hormone therapy from the beginning. Acknowledging Jo's fears, accumulated from reading all those accounts of broken and wrecked marriages due to changes in sexual orientation, I actually waited three months before starting. Then it was only on a quarter dose taking a few more months to get to maximum feminising dosage.

There are two main benefits from hormone therapy. The first to make itself apparent is on the mind. A female brain in a male body awash with testosterone is bad enough, a female brain in a male body trying to become female and awash with testosterone is impossible to live with. As testosterone production was repressed and oestrogen took its place so a peace came about, yet more freedom from that nagging anguish, yet a further step towards feeling complete and whole.

The second benefit is physical. No matter how well I dressed, which normally was horrendously badly in those days, nothing could disguise the contours of my flat boxlike male-developed body. Over time with hormones my shape would change towards those female contours so necessary to pass. Not without its painful bits though, certain changes in shape cause parts of the body to become very sensitive indeed.

Hormones also had another effect. As the oestrogen levels accumulated inside of me I started to have mood swings. I was developing a monthly hormonal mood cycle. For someone not ready to confront an unforeseen effect this was quite unsettling at first and for months it would be very erratic, sometimes happening two or three times a month, sometimes not at all. As time went on it would settle, now it's a regular 28 day cycle but it was certainly something that took a lot of getting used to.

By February Jo and I were beginning to settle down a bit. For all the stresses and emotional hammer blows she had been hit with she was beginning to smile again and beginning to enjoy a life shared with a less anxious, less volatile and far less manic partner. We then had one of those milestones, a totally mundane event, that signalled better things really were on the way.

We had been shopping in London's West End, a normal event for many but for Jo unheard of, shopping with David was hell, an ordeal that in no way ever an event that could be called enjoyable. We had stopped for lunch, they had space heaters outside, we sat outside and people watched. No one was staring at me. We were just an ordinary couple having lunch. We were relaxed and at ease. No longer the raging bull champing to get home, no longer the manic "you've been shopping for 3 ½ minutes, how much longer do you want", no longer "what are we doing wasting time sat here for?", just a normal couple, friends, enjoying each others company on a relaxed weekday afternoon. It had never happened before.

Another notable change, we started going to the theatre together. David occasionally went, under sufferance, always looking at his watch, champing at the bit to get back home but for me it was a whole new thing to enjoy, the occasion, the entertainment and to round the evening off the dinner afterwards in a nice theatre-land restaurant.

However the life of an elegant theatre-going socialite almost fell apart on the first occasion. The show had finished and as we made our way down to the crowded lobby I felt a trip to the loo might be in order as we had a ten minutes walk to the restaurant in front of us. Leaving the loo and making my way back to Jo, oh so elegantly pushing my way through thousands of people, I started to lead her out to the street and accompany her to the restaurant. Jo seemed strangely reluctant to leave and kept whispering something but her serene highness Jennifer was not going to be denied the opportunity for an oh so elegant flaunt through the crowded lobby and became quite insistent that they make a move now.

Jo tried to say something in a whisper but I ignored her knowing I looked such a picture of elegance no one should be denied a glimpse. Jo dragged on my arm, I dragged back, we almost fell to the ground wrestling with each other, then she finally said it, out loud "you stupid tart!! The lining of your skirt is caught up in your knickers!! You are showing all your backside!!" How the mighty are fallen, and not so Oh-so-elegantly fallen either!!

It was time to look at my face. Never a pretty sight at the best of times but male faces built up with all that testosterone are generally so different to female faces some changes are often necessary, in fact in many cases almost total reconstruction is the case, Jawbones being sawn, drilled and ground to different shapes, noses completely reconstructed, large chunks of foreheads removed, ears reshaped, there really is no end. My teeth were awful; there were large bags under my eyes, disfiguring growths there as well. I opted for only a partial rebuild, cowardice deciding a "mature woman" like me does not need a complete rebuild.

Compared to the teeth the eye surgery went pretty smoothly. A few weeks of swollen and bruised eyes and all back to normal again, almost painless The eye bags had been removed but the added bonus was a number of potentially harmful and disfiguring growths had been removed at the same time.

Teeth were a different matter. The only way my upper front teeth would ever be straight is by being removed but I had a phobia about teeth being removed, one of those hangovers from my childhood that no one has ever wanted or dared to try and unearth. Eventually I found the cosmetic dentists who could do the job, who could offer the best possible credentials for being able to do the cosmetic work required, who were willing to work so hard to understand my fears and who could offer the best of care during the procedures including sedation. The days after they completed the first part of the work, even with a temporary bridge in place, would be days of tears as I stared at my smile instead of a disfiguring clump of crooked teeth.

By now the smile was becoming a permanent feature. The often serious David with the crooked teeth rarely smiled, I simply could not give up an opportunity to smile, not just to flash my teeth but to reflect that very profound happiness that was growing inside me.

The teeth also forced something else. In my search for cosmetic dentists who could both do the job and fully accommodate a shivering wreck of a patient resembling

Trapped

wobbly jelly fresh out of a wobbly mould I had finally chosen one who was the other side of London. To drive there would of taken slightly longer than to circumnavigate the globe in a hot air balloon. The London underground could take me straight there but it would be a1½ hour 32 stop journey from one end of the district line to the other. It was time for Jenni's first major solo voyage by public transport. The attempt was meticulously planned, reading material organised, A woman's magazine of the fashion and beauty variety that I could keep my head firmly buried in, quietest carriage, at the front in that compartment where there were only three seats either side of the aisle.

Three stops into this journey and the meticulous planning all fell apart. The train broke down. It was all change. In the melee to get off the magazine was lost. The next train in was crowded, standing room only, it was shoulder to shoulder crushed together sardine fashion, faces two inches apart from each other, no way to avoid eye contact. No one noticed or if they had they never let on. The journey went without incident and another milestone had been passed unlocking yet another door to freedom. Jenni was now free to fly, or at least flaunt herself along the tunnels and platforms of the London underground.

Another journey milestone was driving home on my regular commute from London to Somerset. As more and more people in the small rural community where I lived began to know about my transition so it was time for Jenni to drive herself home. At first I was terrified, I drove half the time with my legs squeezed tightly together as my bladder pleaded with me to obey the call of nature but the fear in my head prevented me from stopping at those large and busy places called service areas.

Then I devised a strategy of stopping at the filling station and rather than have to push my way through a warehouse sized building crowded with people to go into a large and crowded ladies loo I could instead use the small discrete ones at the refuelling area.

Then on one trip home I needed to stop somewhere and do some shopping for dinner. Thank you Marks and Spencer's for on a number of motorway outlets they have now plonked a food shop. With bated breath, praying for holy deliverance and with heart beating at 200 beats per minute I took the plunge. With a full basket I nervously made my way to the counter where my shopping, in the most matter of fact way possible, was put into bags, my charge card charged and without a glimpse of surprise, shock, horror or howls of laughter my card returned with "have a safe drive home Madam." Its now become a routine of mine to pop in on my way home from London, and nearly always its Lorraine, the same member of staff as that first time, who greets me, always the same warm smile, the same genuine interest. Thank you Lorraine, and all your colleagues, you think it's all in a days work, for me it was, well, almost life changing!!

Of great issue was my voice. It was not particularly deep for a male but had loads of chesty resonance. I was often complimented on having a nice speaking voice but now, dressed as a woman, sounding like a bloke with a nice speaking voice was most definitely an unwelcome attribute.

There is no substitute to hard work, patience and sometimes a lot of tears of frustration. Surgery is available to try and raise the pitch of the voice but it is not always successful, in some instances making very little difference, in others making a dramatic difference to the extent the voice that pops out is reminiscent of Minnie mouse on helium.

I decided that a mature 5'10" tall woman would look a bit silly sounding like a sweet, diminutive and demure Minnie mouse. Also it is not only pitch, intonations and rhythms of speech are totally different between male and females. I found the mental image of looking a demure mature female whilst sounding like a bloke trying to imitate mini mouse was just too much for me. It was time for voice training.

There are two parts to that training. The first is learning to raise the voice from out of the chest where it resides with most blokes to the top of the mouth which is where most females talk from. This is part luck and mostly a hell of a lot of practice. I learnt the technique of holding my tongue firm against my back teeth when beginning to speak. I got quite good at it, then went to the dentist who proceeded to rearrange all my teeth so I had to start again. It sometimes took me a bit longer to remember to move my tongue out of the way when starting to speak and a crushed tongue was often the price paid. People got used to hearing me start to speak in ever so sweet and elegant female tones only to watch in horror as my face suddenly contorted with pain and all sorts of gymnastics went on inside my mouth as I tried to talk normal, look normal and find where the hell my tongue was all at the same time.

Intonation was also a difficult problem with me. All too often I found myself talking like a poor imitation of many of the nations favourite drag queens. It took a lot of therapist patience to finally overcome all those inhibitions I had against talking in what to me sounded like a theatrically camp voice.

Holding the pitch is also difficult in stressful situations. Under stress the throat tends to tighten up and the voice slips down a few octaves into that bass resonance so typical of a male. Driving to London one day, in the days when I still had my pose-mobile, a bright red Jaguar XKR convertible with a three digit personalised number plate, I was pulled over by a policeman.

Coming to the passenger side of my vehicle he opened the door and started to give me the nicest telling off I have ever had. Apparently I had committed a slight infringement of the speed limit, not sufficient to warrant a ticket being issued but enough for him to want to pull me over and correct me on my driving. I couldn't help thinking this was a nice way of saying "I'm bored and wanted to see who the smartly dressed bit of totty was driving the posh car with the personalised number plate".

Focussing intently on giving me a professional assessment of my driving skills whilst equally focussed on looking at my legs he finally asked some details, namely name and where I was going to. I flashed my eyelids, gave him my "oh so demure damsel in distress" look, shyly lowered my eyes and through my constricted voice box said "My name is Jennifer, Officer, and I'm on my way to a dinner engagement in London". The voice did not match the rest of the package. I might just of well said "Me name's Fred mate and I'm on me way in to town to have a few pints with me mates". The policeman stared, the look said it all, his ambitions of pulling a smart bit of totty crashed and burned, he mumbled something about driving more carefully in future and sped off in his car leaving the smart bit of totty looking in her vanity mirror contemplating whether she needed a shave that night before going out.

The next issue was my hair. I was taking drugs to help hair growth and hormones themselves were assisting greatly but the old adage of growing hair on a golf ball was proving right. Long flowing locks of beautifully groomed hair look really quite stupid if the mountaintop has an ice-covered plateau, or in my case if a beautifully smooth and glistening dome of saucer-sized shaped baldness appeared above the sides of cascading tresses.

I tried every alternative I could find. One alternative that was unacceptable was wearing a wig. One thing is they are too restrictive, there are just two many things I could not do with a wig that would of made the permanent wearing of one intolerable. The other was wigs have a habit of coming off at the most inconvenient of times and they are particularly susceptible to high winds. I lost count of the number of times I found myself walking down a busy high street with my mobile phone pressed firmly against my ear, when in actual fact I was grabbing hold of my flowing tresses. On really windy days two mobile phones held to both ears would have to be resorted to, either that or not go out at all, and even for all my irrepressible joy at being out and free the thought of walking along with a phone held firmly to each ear would be just too much. Those days were days when it was time to stay in and indulge in a spot of flat-cleaning.

I tried everywhere to find the hair replacement or augmentation system that would give me the freedom I so desired but also would give me the feeling of naturalness and of femininity. Finally, just like with the dentist, the right people came along.

This company offered tailor made individual systems crafted to the individual need. By blending with the contours and hair growing patterns of my natural hair and using a mix of bonding techniques I could end up with something that looked and felt natural, felt part of me, would allow me total unrestricted freedom of movement. I could take a shower or go swimming with no worries, I could groom, style and colour however I wanted and walk down the high street in gale force winds without having a battery of mobile phones held firmly to my ears. It was to be another major step in transition, the feeling of freedom and natural femininity that flowed just made me feel so warm and whole inside. The transition from him to her was approaching completion.

The process of coming out to people that at first appeared to progress so dreadfully slowly accelerated as confidence grew and then finally we reached the end of the list of people to tell. It was fortuitous timing. As the list of people who knew of the changes grew and grew so did the risks of it becoming public knowledge and gossip. The week we told the last person on our list, the last person we wanted to tell before it became grapevine gossip, the news leaked out into the small community where we lived.

Now there were to be no secrets, no hiding. I could now change all my documents. Driver's license was changed to tell the traffic police I was a female driver, tax records was changed so I could pay tax as a female citizen of the state and my medical records were changed to record the fact I was now female even if it did mean declining the invitation for a cervical smear scan.

The big day though was the day I went to collect my new passport. My appointment was for 12-o-clock and after queuing for just 10 minutes outside at just before noon I was allowed into the building, cleared security and then nervously waited to be called. I didn't wait long; then, even more nervously I made my way to the counter; a very helpful official checked all my documents before disappearing into a huddle with his colleague. His colleague, a lovely smiling lady came over after a few minutes and said "OK Miss Brown, take this voucher to the cash desk, pay the fee and exactly four hours after that you can collect your new passport".

I collected my receipt with the time stamp on it, had four hours to kill so dashed off to Oxford Street to have my ears pierced. He had only pierced one ear when my phone rang. Something told me it was the passport office, "do you mind?" I asked giving the piercing man no choice as I got out of the chair and rushed to my bag to retrieve my phone. It was the passport office, they had forgotten to ask for my birth certificate, "Be right back" I shouted to the astonished piercing man and dashed out and hastily flagged down a taxi to take me back to the passport office, one ear pierced and the other still with a bit of tape attached to it.

Security clearly had some sympathy with the breathless woman with one pierced ear, cleared me to go to the counter straight away, the same lovely smiling woman took my birth certificate, "Everything seems ok, same time as on your receipt, possibly a few minutes late". A dash back to Oxford street, muttered apologies to the piercing man who seemed to pierce my other ear with quite a sadistic grin on his face, then back to wait in the collection part. Finally my name called, "Miss Brown to position 2".

"Can you check the details please Ma'am" said the woman; I looked only at one line, "Yes that's ok" handing my passport back. She looked at me a little quizzically before handing it back to me with "I mean can you take a few minutes and check all the details?" she asked. "That's ok" I said handing it back, She started to hand it back to me again, noticed the tears streaming down my face, softly read all the details back to me, I nodded my confirmation they were all correct, "are you ok?" She asked with gentle concern, "Yes, its just that one line, means so much to me" I sniffled back, "Oh, what line is that" She asked, "The line where it says "Sex" and then has an "F" against it" I blubbered. She smiled, understood what I had been saying, handed me my nice shiny new passport with the words "welcome to the start of your new life Miss Brown". So lovely, they all were, the passport office all the way through from my original telephone call to discuss procedure showed a kindness and compassion rare in so many places. Thank you all.

Having that passport in my handbag changed my life. One thing to have a driver's license with a female face staring out of it and "Miss Jennifer" on the name line but the passport says unequivocally "Female". All of a sudden I could hold myself straighter, look more people in the eye, and have a hundred percent more confidence in myself. It didn't matter now what other people thought, here was the proof that as far as the state was concerned I was legally and medically considered to be female.

As my year of real life test came to a close I felt an inner confidence grow, I was dressing better, laborious sessions of voice coaching and hours of practice had feminised my voice, or at least removed the worst of the "maleness", the pain and trauma of massive dental reconstruction, not just those hideous upper front teeth had given me the confidence to smile, I was not only dressing better but with my shoe problems resolved I was also walking better, my physical shape was changing, inside I felt more feminine, more free, more liberated, more me.

A time came, possibly almost on the anniversary of that first trip to the supermarket, that first trip of such apprehensive nervousness when I had made my first solo journey as Jenni, a solo trip made with my face caked with screen foundation, multiple shades of blusher, and three contrasting shades of eye shadow all set off with lipstick that matched none of the rest of that gorgeous kaleidoscope of feminine allure.

I was preparing a supper for a group of people that were meeting at my home. I had run out of a couple of things. Taking my apron off, hair still tied back, not a splash of make-up on, I dashed over to the local supermarket. My development age had now matured to that of an elegant, sophisticated and vibrantly youthful mid-30's woman, well, in my dreams it had, and the nearly flat sensible shoes, calf length skirt and comfortable baggy top reflected my youthful elegance. I Stopped on the way to have a quick chat to a friend I bumped into and on the way back popped into the local beauticians to make an appointment for some bits and pieces to be done. I remembered about some long-forgotten laundry, spare bedding, I had left in a local launderer and made a short detour to collect it, having a laugh and a joke with the proprietor about having forgotten it and what would of happened if I had unexpected visitors. I returned home and it struck me the change that had taken place in just one year. I knew then, I had passed the test, I had finished transition, I was me, Jenni Brown - female.

Chapter 12
Now

So, where are Jo and I now?

I suppose from my point of view I can say definitely I have transitioned, or at least transitioned enough that I can now live a perfectly normal life as a female. Transitioning will never ever stop, I know it is a continuous process that will be with me until I die but at least now I am comfortable. Gender Reassignment Surgery is still something waiting to happen, or at least awaiting a decision on whether it will go ahead or not. I have all the letters of referral, have seen the surgeon and have had appointments for a bed booked but it is dependent on other factors involving issues outside of my control to be resolved first. I have not discussed those other issues in this book. They are issues that affect me deeply, could have a profound effect on my future whatever happens and alone they could form a whole chapter, and as and when a final decision is taken then probably that will signal an updating, I did say in the introduction that this book can be considered a version 1!!

It is fundamentally important to me. Without it I will never be complete, always have part of the jigsaw missing.

Without it happening I will always feel as though I am living a lie, what's inside the packet being different to what's described on the label. If I had to try and establish some form of measurement I would say I feel only 75% complete without it but that does not mean I cannot live without it. If I was to continue with the hypothetical scale of measurement I would say that prior to transition I must of only been 25% complete, my life, my happiness, my confidence, my knowledge of who and what I am now has so fundamentally improved that if I stayed as I was then I would be for ever grateful transition has happened despite all the pain and sacrifice, but that missing piece would always be a hole that without being filled will render the remainder an incomplete picture.

I don't "pass" in the sense I can go through life without it ever being noticed that I was once something else. 40 years of adult male behaviour does not get overridden that easily, a careless slouch of the shoulders, a swagger of the arms, a drop of the head, the wrong profile accentuating my testosterone-sculptured face are all give-aways as is the dropping of pitch in the voice or the wrong lilt at the end of sentences when I get careless. However there is a big difference between not passing and not being acceptable and most people now accept me as just another female, ok one who may sometimes be a bit different, who's physical body may not always have been typically female, but nonetheless someone who is female.

Jo and I have had to resolve many personal issues regarding our relationship with each other. Jo is heterosexual and as feminising physical changes started to take place with me she felt that as a heterosexual female she could no longer share a bed with someone who now also had very obvious female characteristics. This is just one of the many issues we have had to resolve together but it has in no way diminished the love that is between us or the affection we both hold for each other. Indeed in many ways it has enhanced our relationship in that we now are far more open and honest with each other, there are no secrets, there are no issues going unmentioned for fear of hurting each other and this openness and honesty between us has given back in different ways so much of what we could of lost.

I am still getting used to that lack of anguish inside. Contentment is a strange thing. Try and describe it to someone, I still keep waiting for the internal bomb to go off and still have not got used to the fact that it is now defused. Another word it is almost impossible to describe is "normal", but that is how I feel, normal, not out of step anymore, not dislocated with my peer group, not confused as to what I should be doing, not afraid to show what I thought others would see as inappropriate feminine responses, I just simply feel totally normal. If I heard someone shout out the word "freak" or "tranny" in the street now I would look around to see who they were saying that to, it simply no longer applies to me.

I smile a lot more, without exception people who knew both presentations say I am so much more relaxed, nicer to be with, less intense, less serious Even now sometimes I will be walking down the street and it will suddenly hit me, a feeling of freedom and liberation that still makes my head swim and cause an involuntary smile to stretch from ear to ear. My awareness of my surroundings has become a joy. When I am out, which is the majority of the time, I notice more, smell more, hear birds singing, spend far more time looking at different things, in different shop windows, as if giving myself just that little bit more time to do things, not to be in so much of a hurry, has actually heightened my senses.

In sharp contrast to my childhood my adult life has always been gregarious, sometimes exhaustingly so. Jo and I always had many friends, were always socialising, and were always getting involved in a variety of activities and interests. My fear with transition was that could well dry up. It hasn't, if anything our lifestyle is now even more active and gregarious now and for me immeasurably more pleasurable as I no longer feel that nagging need to hold a discussion with intense passion or to organise every single event with complete military precision, often throwing a wobbly whenever anyone dared break with the plan or programme, I mean, How dare they enjoy themselves at the expense of my meticulous planning?. Now, its let things happen as they happen, I still like to be organised, will still nag over the detail, but organisation is only the means to facilitate an event, its not the event itself and if things don't go to plan sometimes it's no big deal any more.

I still have a great passion for the under-privileged and hate to see people bullied or abused, be it children or physically or mentally weaker adults but no longer do I feel the need to go off on one and single-handed try and change the world. I am much more measured now. I still have traits of that obsessive behaviour but nothing like the self-destruct intensity that was so prevalent when I was David. There is no longer the danger of throwing myself into a cause with a passion leading to over-commitment because I simply do not want to get that involved, I am much more prepared now to delegate, let others better equipped than me worry about issues, I will let my writing do the talking as and when I can be bothered to write!!

Like that child of so many years ago I cry easily. Now though I don't have to choke back my tears. I can learn of the horrors of Dafur in Western Sudan as they unfold, hear of animals being abused, watch the news as terrible stories of abused and neglected children are broadcast and I don't need to hold it all back like David had to, I can just go ahead and cry and welcome the release of my tears. Sometimes I feel David's compassion, feel his anger and imagine what it must have been like for him not to have been able to express that release. It is little wonder the intensity with which his compassion and anger found a release in other, often self-destructive, ways.

A very strange feeling I have is that all my male adult years have been stripped away, eradicated as though they never really existed. I am in a continuum with that child and as that child used to pray very simply to God for peace and comfort so it was as though God took that child, when it was ready to grow up, and led it along that path of growing up but not as David, as Jenni. As I say in my chapter on faith there was no Jenni until I had found my faith again and it was only once I had returned to that faith, a faith I put on the back-burner when I entered my adult years, that I was allowed to grow into the adult I was intended to be.

Something else had to go, Alcohol. Apart from anything else a huge beer belly is not the most desirable of feminine shapes, I would prefer to have curves somewhere else. However life now is too good to waste it by ruining my health through excessive drinking. Almost as soon as the strain of transition started to ease and the joy of just being Jenni was allowed to start to fully shine through so the need for alcohol started to abate. However it had become a habit if not an addiction and like any habit was going to prove hard to break but It had to be broken. I have not forsaken alcohol altogether, I like my glass of wine, but no way am I ever going to return to that routine of drinking every day, opening another bottle of wine after dinner, carrying yet another bottle of wine upstairs to my office every time I was digging in to work late. Life now is just too good, too beautiful, to waste on alcohol abuse and now I just have no need for it anyway. Dare I say it? Life for the first time is now worth living for.

One thing that has not gone, sadly, is facial hair. I remark in my transition chapter the need for either painful electrolysis or almost equally painful but far quicker laser depilation. Laser was very successful in removing the thickest growths and the darkest of hair removing both vigorous growth and a beard shadow and in turn also removing the need for thick concealing make-up. However since finishing laser treatment the hair growth has restarted, albeit much finer and white, not dark, but I still have to start a lengthy and painful course of electrolysis to remove the growth permanently.

In fact this is the one shadow I have on my life now. A small, slight shadow but still a bit of a downer is the need every week for further on-going painful treatments. After nearly three years of it I want a break if nothing else and now facial electrolysis is not only necessary, so is electrolysis in other regions as part of pre-surgery preparations. It's no big deal and something I know will bear hugely worthwhile rewards in the future but I would not be human if every so often I did not mutter "Give me a break" under my breath as I left home for yet more painful treatment somewhere.

As for Jo?

I will not speak for her; I will let her tell her own story in her own chapter. I do see her now just starting to believe she is at last escaping from that long dark tunnel. A tunnel that started 20 years ago with all those fears over her husbands health only to see him recover and disappear all over the world then return and at a time she probably needed a lot of tender loving care so he was spending 20 hours a day caring for everyone else. Then her son running off to the USA in a bizarre and fretful relationship, her life being turned upside down by moving from a home she was so settled and happy in, the terrible accident to her son in the United States then the devastation of 18 policemen searching every corner of her home. Living through all that terrible misleading and inciting press coverage, supporting her husband through the aftermath only to find she was now living with an unpredictable volatile tornado, the pain and hurt of thinking that after all that unconditional and unflinching support and love she had shown she was now being cheated on as her husband shared his life with another woman only then to find out there was another woman but it was her husband and he was about to be she.

I cry as I type these words. The only thing I want for Jo now is a huge share of my new-found peace and contentment to flow to her, to see her smile again, to feel secure again, to feel safe and loved again. God bless you Jo, god bless the woman I love so much, my wife, my partner for life, my best friend and soul mate, God bless you. I love you.

Chapter 13
Jo's story

Before I say anything about David, Jenni or myself, I want to say first and foremost that this tale would in all likelihood have had a completely different ending without the committed love and support of so many friends and family. They have shared my tears, made me laugh and no words of thanks can express my gratitude. Thanks also go to my animals who gave me a reason to keep going when the going got tough.

My deepest gratitude is to Jesus - for everything!

Life with David was akin to living on Blackpool's famous Big Dipper, life now with Jen is like living on a gentle carousel!

David has explained how we came to meet each other. For my part I was extremely attracted to this funny, highly intelligent and very macho man. He was so interesting on virtually any subject. Any knowledge he gained, he retained, his brain-power was phenomenal and he was an extremely stimulating person to be with. Our sense of humour matched, and we spent hours laughing about anything and everything. Life was fun!

Although not as tall as the man I'd always envisaged marrying, he was all man - no effeminate streak at all, and I knew this was the man I wanted to spend the rest of my life with. If only I'd known what lay ahead!

Our first years together were hard. We both worked to capacity and as well as work, had twin boys to cope with. We had very little money, and we ended each day exhausted

Throughout our married life we have moved house nine times. Twice for my job in the early years as a Warden of an old peoples sheltered housing scheme, and six times for David's job. We moved from Manchester to Preston, Surrey, Bristol, Lancashire and Somerset, then to where we live now. The last move was because I wanted to.

I am quite boring in some ways, and one of those ways is that my home has always been important to me. But it always felt that as soon as I'd got my house in some sort of order, made new friends, settled the boys into school, the ever-restless David would instigate yet another move. I felt constantly uprooted. The upside to all this moving was that as David's career progressed, each house was nicer than the last.

Looking back on our early years, David was a typical husband and father. He was ecstatic when the twins were born, so proud! Unusually for men all those years ago, he was happy to share with childcare, night feeds, nappy changes etc. Although life was tough, we were very happy, and I felt blessed.

The hardest thing for me to cope with in our marriage was David's often irrational behaviour. His sudden temper tantrums, inexplicable rages and overbearing attitude were difficult to bear. I was forever trying to keep the peace, anticipate possible trigger points and attempt to reason with him, never with any real success. However, I rationalised that David worked incredibly long hours, and put his mood swings down to pressure of work.

Trapped

As the boys grew, David tried to be the best father he could, given his heavy work commitments. He tried to get the boys interested in football, rock climbing and all the usual boys' pursuits. Whenever possible, he attended school events, Parents' Evenings, and took an interest in the boys schooling and homework.

Still, life with David was never easy, mainly due to his manic lifestyle. He worked long hours, often off on business trips, I was left to cope with the boys, and life could be lonely at times. When he was home, every minute had to be filled with frantic activity. He could never sit down and relax. However, we muddled through as best we could, and our family life seemed normal, and ordinary, and much the same as everyone else's.

Due to oxygen deprivation at birth, Adam had slight learning difficulties and it was not until we moved to this area that this was recognised and he received specialist help. Until then he had struggled in mainstream schools. At his Special Needs School, his education progressed in leaps and bounds and I will never cease to be grateful for that school.

In time Adam left school and embarked on a series of training schemes, none of which suited. By this time he was living in a nearby town, and Jenni has described his subsequent hasty marriage to Tolly, and then his serious micro light accident in which he lost four fingers.

David was feeling restless once more, and suggested a move to America. I really did not want to go, I felt happy with my home, family and friends here. David can be very persuasive! He pointed out the improved lifestyle we would have, and the better climate. He was willing to ship over my animals. Bit by bit he chipped away at my reluctance, but I finally agreed when I realised we would be closer to Adam, who we felt really needed our support at this difficult time.

So we were in the process of this move when the phone call came from David's secretary, a call that turned our lives upside down.

At first I was not too worried about the police raids on our London flat and our country home. I'd heard of people who download internet pornography and of paedophiles who abuse children. After all, for many years now I'd had to listen to David's anger and experience his zealous crusade against these people. I truly believed this was a misunderstanding that could easily be cleared up with the police. They were only doing their job, but somehow they had targeted the wrong person. I almost felt sorry for them and the apology they would have to make once they realised David's views on child pornography, paedophiles, and the efforts he had made to help victims of childhood abuse in particular. There was enough documented evidence of this, so many people that David had helped, including the police themselves, who could testify on his behalf. All the police had to do was make a few enquiries, and they would quickly see their mistake.

So confident was I that this would quickly be resolved that we almost booked our return tickets to Virginia when we set off from Washington. Just how naive I was being, very quickly became apparent. The nightmare was just beginning of what was to become the darkest days of my life. Nothing would ever be the same again.

We arrived back home to find that no less than 18 police officers had invaded our home, inspected all our personal possessions and removed the PC's (which incidentally, despite an order from a Judge have never been returned to us).

Far from the apology we had expected, the Police regarded us as guilty from Day One. David was treated as though guilty of the most horrendous things. Nothing he could say could persuade them of his innocence. I began to feel very, very frightened.

Word quickly spread amongst our small community. I felt that I did not want to leave our home, to face the stares of people who must have believed David to be guilty of the most heinous crimes. This is just about the worst thing to accuse anyone of, anything related to the abuse of children, yet no attempt was ever made by either the press or police to disclose the true nature of what he was being accused of. I knew that David was innocent. Had I believed for one second it could be true, I would not have felt able to stand by my husband. I just felt powerless to help him.

Whilst I did not want to leave home, I did not feel safe at home either. The picture that was being publicly painted was that this was a man who delighted in viewing images of children being abused! I feared vigilante attacks on us, our property and our animals. I could not sleep at night, I could only pray to God that this nightmare would soon be over and our lives could go back to normal.

Luckily God must have been listening! Over the coming weeks and months, friends, family and neighbours offered their endless love and support. We could not have got through this without them. I felt that my prayers had been answered and a miracle had taken place in that we were never attacked, neither verbally or physically.

All that needed to happen now was for the truth to come out so that David could be completely exonerated, and to have his reputation restored.

David has described the subsequent investigation and how it went so badly wrong. You hear about "miscarriages of justice" all the time, but when it is happening to the man you love, nothing can describe the powerlessness this brings. I watched David's life unravel before my eyes and could do nothing to stop it. My only strength came through prayer, something I relied on more and more.

As we'd had so much support from the church and community and no adverse reactions, we decided to stay in the village. Luckily the house sale had not gone through, so we sold the house in Virginia, and tried to get our lives back on track.

If only life could be that simple! David became unbearable to live with. He was filled with anger and rage at the injustice that had been done. I tried to understand. Over the next few years things got only worse. He would fly off into a temper at the drop of a hat. I like a calm life, and tried as best I could to diffuse his rages, but he would turn on me with angry, hurtful words that broke my heart again and again.

By this time David was spending more and more time in London. We were leading increasingly separate lives. It seemed like he could not bear to be around me. More than once he drove home from London to spend the weekend here, only to storm out immediately and drive all the way back because of something I said - or did not say! It was impossible to know what I was doing wrong, or what would trigger off the next outburst.

Life was intolerable. I began to make new friends, take up new interests, but this only widened the gap between us. Then strange things happened. Letters and parcels began to arrive for "Miss Jenni Brown" I never opened them, just put them on David's desk. I never asked about them, and he never offered any explanation. I would walk into his office and he would look guilty, obviously trying to hide something on screen from me. He'd already told me he had another flat in London, but would not tell me where, said he needed a "bolt hole". Slowly I began to add up all the pieces, David's absences and his indifference to me, his rages. It was all so obvious, he had got Another Woman.

I felt betrayed. After All I had Done for Him! My life had been turned upside down by David's manic obsession with "Justice for the World", the "Righting of Wrongs" for the underprivileged, the poor, the homeless, the abused. Where was the gratitude I deserved for standing by him and believing in him? Now David had found himself a newer model, and I was to be cast aside like an old overcoat

Trapped

that now longer fitted. I hated Miss Jenni Brown with a vengeance!

At the same time I felt very jealous of her. Obviously she did not see the hurtful person that David had become with me. She had the happy, funny and intelligent David that I used to have. David's pathetic excuse of needing a bolt hole was a lie. Clearly it was a Love Nest that he shared with Miss Jenni Brown!

I still loved David. He was my best friend and I wanted the old David back. I hoped this would be a fling that would run its' course, so I said nothing. Like countless other women in this position I buried my head in the sand and prayed for this to go away.

I did not want my marriage to end, but at the same time was not willing to fight for someone who could treat me so shabbily. I began to wonder how my life would be without David to look after me. I turned my thoughts to how I could survive alone, and considered ways in which I could turn our home into a B&B. I felt destabilised and resentful. Far from missing David's company, I was relieved to spend more time without him. Life was more peaceful without the rows, anger and sulks I'd have to endure when he was here. No, I was better off without him. Miss Jenni Brown was welcome to him!

Sometimes though we would have surprising and unexpected periods of calm, when things would be more like the old times, we'd even share laughter! It was during one of these relaxed times that David dropped his latest bombshell into my lap. On 1st July I found out that there was indeed a Miss Jenni Brown sharing David's life, and that Miss Jenni Brown was in fact my husband!

We had recently heard that an elderly uncle of mine had been "outed" as a cross-dresser. I was curious, but felt upset for him about the ridicule he was receiving. David and I talked about this, and I said I felt it was nobody's business but his, it was harmless. David could not let the subject drop, and returned to it constantly. "Did I really feel this way?"; "Don't I think it a bit odd?" Eventually I couldn't resist asking, with a laugh, "Have you ever tried this?" Nothing on earth could have prepared me for the reply I received.

Gently David explained to me about Gender Dysphoria. As the words soaked into my brain, I felt an overriding feeling of relief. There was no other woman; my faith in David had not been misplaced. Suddenly David's behaviour began to make sense. I felt David's pain and isolation and just wanted to hug him for sharing this difficult news with me. I wanted to help.

In those days I knew nothing about Gender Dysphoria. I'd heard of men who dressed as women and assumed it was some sexual aberration. Transsexuals – transvestites – all the same to me. It had no bearing or interest in my life. I did suffer some jealousy of the people in London with whom David had shared this part of his life, I suppose I felt excluded. All this time I'd been kept in ignorance, while David had confided in others and had relied on their support.

I turned to the internet for information. I was completely overwhelmed by what I found. Of course I read the worst possible scenarios, how hormones could affect ones sexuality, how full transition could leave the woman seeking a male partner. I worried endlessly. I have left it to David to give an explanation of Gender Dysphoria and its' implications.

We had many heart to heart discussions on where we should go from here. David suggested divorce, he could not envisage my acceptance or support. With our rediscovered closeness, I felt we could work something out. I did not want to lose David, even if it meant I had to have Jenni in my life. I had fallen in love with this person, my soul mate and best friend, and this person was still there, albeit with a new identity.

I still did not realise the full implications of what Gender Dysphoria meant. I initially thought that David would need to be Jenni for 40% of the time to feel comfortable. The remaining 60% of the time, I could have my husband back, I felt I could just about cope with that.

However, it soon became very clear to me that there was no choice for David, only becoming Jenni 100% could ever be acceptable. I had much to learn. It was time to meet Miss Jenni Brown in person!

We agreed that I would go up to London and meet Jenni at the flat, and we would go out for a meal together. On the long, hot journey up I kept telling myself "just accept it… just accept it." over and over again, like a mantra.

Nothing could have prepared me for my first sight of Jenni. She answered the door wearing a long wig held in place with glitter clips, a black silk blouse, red mini skirt and black stockings. "Tranny" shoes completed the glorious ensemble! Now I have always been a very conservative dresser. I had tried my best to understand the Jenni thing, and here I was, on a hot summers' evening, being expected to go out in public, for dinner in a posh restaurant, with someone who looked like a prostitute! We sat at the back of the restaurant, and all I could feel was acute embarrassment! The very next day we went straight to M&S for a change of wardrobe!

We now entered a strange period of limbo in which for various reasons, mostly his own denial, David would return back to being himself but when he did this the depression it caused led to violent mood swings which I found intolerable. Eventually it reached a stage where I had to make my feelings known quite strongly and to cut a long story short David finally agreed to undergo medical transition. Now at last our new life could begin: a life with only Jenni.

Originally I found excursions into the big outside world with Jenni to be quite embarrassing. I am a shy, reserved person, not comfortable with people looking at me and now I found myself in the company of someone who attracted a lot of stares for the wrong reasons. Then I would found myself becoming quite protective of her which then gave me courage and strength to be with her.

Jenni's hormone treatment made it feel like I was living with a pubescent teenager! Her Prima Donna flounces were legendary! But unlike with David, you could easily turn Jenni's sulks and tantrums into laughter! Though I have effectively lost David, having Jenni in my life is so much fun! It's like having a beloved sister living here. She is so relaxed and we enjoy each others' company. While I would never say that I am glad all these terrible things have happened to bring Jenni into my life, I am not sorry either!

This adjustment period when Jenni was still looking sadly like a man dressing as a woman seemed to go on forever but now looking back it passed quite quickly. After a few months it began to dawn on me that being out in public with Jenni was no longer attracting unwelcome attention, she was rarely getting noticed, being taken most of the time as just another woman. Now I felt I could begin to relax and properly get to know this new person in my life.

Jenni occasionally reverts back to being David in terms of volatile temperament but now life is much calmer, more relaxed and I can now feel as though I can share my feelings and my concerns more freely and openly. We laugh more together and as Jenni matures she can laugh at herself more, her initial preciousness about her appearance is now giving way to humorous self-deprecation. I also feel as though I have more input into our joint lives, where David was always travelling at 120 miles an hour and leaving everyone else behind in the process Jenni is calmer, more relaxed and far more ready to listen.

I now feel as though I am emerging from that long dark tunnel. I don't want David back!!. Life is far more fun with my big Sister Jen.

Chapter 14
Faith

In chapter 10 I describe how looking in that mirror, being re-united with that child of so long ago, was like all my adult years disappearing and a continuum with all those feelings of dislocation and being different in my childhood being established.

So it was too with my faith.

As a child I was not brought up to be religious, Mum had a simple faith, encouraged her children to believe and go to church sometimes, Dad thought it was "all a load of old cobblers" and praying and believing in god was somehow something "not manly".

I often prayed to God, very simply, almost as if in discussion with an older wiser friend, A place that always sticks in my mind is a small park near the prefab that for the first 12 years of my life was home. This park consisted mostly of large ornamental trees and shrubs and in one part a half circle had been cut into and lined with three park benches as a place for people to meet and gossip the day away. Behind these benches was a thicket of large laurel and rhododendron bushes and it was there I used to go sometimes, spending hours hidden away from view, a place of peace and solitude and somewhere I often talked to God.

As I moved into adulthood I lost that faith, it wasn't a "manly" thing to profess anyway and everything I did had to be manly and macho. In May of that awful year, during those shattering months of being investigated, I had a very strange experience. I was in London and found myself walking around that small park, the half circle of benches still there and a strange feeling of being united with my childhood sweeping over me. Even stranger, I had no recollection of getting there, no memory of waking up, getting dressed, catching the underground to travel across West London or the ten minute walk from the station. It was as though someone was taking me back to those days when in my distressed and anguished world I would appeal to God for help, almost as if someone was taking me out of an adulthood full of denial, suppression and non-belief back to where I had left off as a child, a child desperate to find out who he really was and with a simple faith to carry him through the trials of travelling that journey of realisation..

Jo is a Christian and an active member of our local church. A couple of months after this strange event and there was a meeting of all the church home groups on our rear terrace. Despite weather forecasts to the contrary it was a dry sunny evening. I had that week had a meeting with my solicitor that was less than encouraging. My stomach was churning and the weight of the investigation was making me seriously concerned that I might even be losing mental control. I felt a presence. A feeling of calm and peace came over me. I had been re-united with my childhood faith and now knew a greater authority than government and the criminal justice service was on my side. God's judgement was the one that mattered, not the judgements of flawed and mortal men. I became a Christian. With me at least there was no training course or apprenticeship or learning curve

Trapped

to faith. That day my faith became absolute, my conviction in Jesus and my love for God unshakeable. What I didn't know then was that as well as becoming "born again" as a Christian, I was also going to become "Born-again" as a person..

The first stage in my journey of growing up was being taken back to my place of solitude as a child, looking back now with the benefit of hindsight and the knowledge of a lot of unrelated events that now fuse together I can now see that God was taking me back to when I believed, had faith and showed it in simple prayer. My new life was to begin from there and in doing so it eradicated all those years when I had moved away from his side, all those adult years of painful anguish and explosive and manic over-commitment.

Reunited with God my unshakeable faith in him and in my belief that in the end it was his judgement that mattered carried me through those terrible last months of that year. As those grossly inaccurate headlines were carried on the front page of the local press I felt God's protection. Our local church family were magnificent through those times and afterwards, never wavering in their love, belief and unconditional support. Then, two years later, when they were to learn that David was now Jenni, it was the same again, unequivocal love.

The end of that year, as recounted in my emergence chapter, that pubescent child inside, a continuation of that child that was abandoned by me as I entered adulthood, began to emerge. Sat on my bed in my run-down flat that was awaiting refurbishment my pleas and prayers were answered. My cries for an answer, an answer to why my adult life had been such a progression of slamming into brick walls were answered and as always, were answered suddenly and forcefully. No dawning of realisation, no gradual emergence, the answer was clear, loud and unequivocal, I was the wrong way round and my growth as the true person within was now going to begin, to restart from that time I abandoned my faith and that child. That, as recounted in chapter 10, was the first time in my adult life I felt a need to present myself as female.

I recount in my chapter on emergence how with faltering steps that female persona emerged, how she was given her name, how she matured and finally how revulsion at this sleazy unnatural behaviour forced David to abandon her in October of that year, an action that was to plunge him into the gravest crisis of his life. A month before, in September, yet another strange event was to occur that was to leave me puzzled for months, years even.

My coming out, my emergence as Jenni, had in those early months been faltering steps within a fetish community. That Summer I had agreed to be hostess of a "munch", a regular social event of like-minded friends meeting in a pub. The pub chosen was a large establishment with a rather fine beer garden on Chiswick High Road in London.

The September munch was a bit of a fiasco. The landlord had double-booked two events and our event was consigned to the garden. Inside a 21st birthday party was in full swing and I was soon chatting to many of the revellers who suggested we join them and have just one big party. It was a cold September evening so this suggestion was greeted with enthusiasm and the garden emptied as we all trooped in.

I then had an overwhelming feeling propelling me back out into the solitude of that garden. I felt no cold as I went outside. I prayed. A feeling of peace and calm swept over me and I knew the Holy Spirit of our Father was with me. I felt his love wash over me. It was an astounding, awesome experience.

The following month David, beset with feelings of guilt and self-loathing, drove Jenni from his mind and almost immediately he was plunged into grave crisis as his mind went into turmoil. Gone was his rock, his anchor of being

Trapped

the person he truly was but the person he couldn't accept, Instead it was back to that churning anguish of his adulthood, only this time the person inwardly he knew was false.

For nine months a desperate struggle was to rage inside his mind, a life and death struggle for as his mental strength weakened and became exhausted so he was beset by almost overwhelming feelings towards self-destruction. One of the most compulsive episodes was on the platform at Hammersmith Underground station, a sudden compulsion to throw himself on the rails and be free from all that incredibly painful and corrosive anguish, his feet rocking on the platform edge he felt a tug on his right shoulder, someone was making him walk backwards from that edge. There was no one, not in the mortal sense, but when the tugging stopped he was staring at a flight of steps and a sign that said "Exit".

It was my faith that carried me through the worst of those terrible times but what was that episode in September about? I now see it clearly. At that time I was presenting as Jenni about 30% of the time, David the remaining 70%. God, aware of the trials coming up, sent a message, a message reminding me of his presence, a message that my faith was not misplaced. It was a message to continue to believe despite all the horrors that were to come to me, to have faith and all will come right. He sent this message to Jenni, not to David. Despite the fact I was David for a large majority of the time the message came to me as Jenni, God was showing his love for me. This is the only explanation my head can arrive at, my heart needs no explanation.

As stated elsewhere in this book, I am an emotional person. Always, when I have felt the love and support of his Holy Spirit beside me my tears have flowed, the same tears that would fall from the eyes of a child when comforted and supported by a loving father putting his strong protective arms around that child.

The time came for Jenni to go to church. At long last I felt strong enough to walk into a church on my own, kneel and pray and receive Holy Communion. Needless to say my presence caused some to stare, but not in a malicious way, just with the curiosity I know I must expect to attract. Soon though they had another reason to stare. The tears would not stop flowing, as I stood to sing in worship so my whole body just shuddered with internal relief and feelings of overwhelming love. There was nothing I could do to stop it and throughout that service it would not stop. The feeling I had of God's arms around me was just so huge, so overwhelming, it was the embrace a Father reserves for a long lost child coming home. I was home.

Now, living full time as Jenni I find myself so welcomed by so many Christian communities. I say Communities for it's not necessarily true of the Christian establishment. One of the biggest opponents of the Gender Recognition Act which came into force in 2004 and gave people such as myself restoration of many of our human rights was the evangelical alliance. They seem to believe that my salvation of being able to live my life in the form that God made me would be to embrace the teachings and love of Jesus Christ.

There we have a problem for it was only when I opened my heart up to God, when I felt the love of Jesus Christ, I started to exist, Jenni was able to escape from her prison and a lifetime of churning anguish and pain was able to end. Perhaps they believe I have faith in a false God, that it was the devil I listened to, the devil that carried me through all that turmoil, the devil that saved me from self-destruction and the devil that returned me safely to God. Perhaps they even believe that they know better than God. Perhaps God has made a mistake, perhaps when I embraced God with all my heart and all my soul and he shined his love upon me as Jenni he should of waited until I had changed back into that person full of pain and churning anguish, the person they know is the right person. If only God would listen to them and not expect them to listen to him I might of got it right.

Needless to say the assumption that I am an abomination to God and that everyone else including God has got it wrong also depends on the assumption that all the results of scientific studies and the conclusions of medical and psychological analysis must be wrong as well. If after all they even had a grain of truth in them we would all have to accept that I am as God made me, someone with the brain of a female and the body of a male. If that was the case then surely I honour God with my brain, the place where my mind and soul lives, not my genitals, so do I obey the will of my mind or live with the flaws of my body?

Sadly it is not only the evangelical alliance with who I appear to be in conflict.

My local church family, as represented by the congregation of my local parish church, stood by me firmly during and after the events of that terrible period of police investigation. The love shown was both immeasurable and invaluable. During all that period they defied the glare of publicity by using my home as a venue for many meetings. In the years that followed my home continued to be used both for church community purposes and also to host widely publicised Alpha Courses which I also took part in leading. Alpha is an important evangelical tool explaining in simple ways the principles of the Christian church. I also provided for church fundraising events to be held in other locations and took part in helping a neighbouring parish with its alpha course. The only time my involvement in the church was questioned was when my name was proposed to the diocese to be a synod representative for the parish at diocese meetings and senior figures questioned whether someone so recently involved in an investigation involving so much odious publicity should be the representative.

Then when my transition became public it all changed. Suddenly I was an unacceptable face of the Christian church. Not only was I made a pariah, my home, a home that up until then had publicly been used for high profile events like alpha, that surely must of been used with the knowledge of all concerned at all levels right up to the diocese administration, was put off limits for all church functions. My wife herself was forbidden to host church events at our home even if I gave a solemn undertaking not to be there.

The church assures me this is in response to the events of that police action and the aftermath that followed and they are not practicing gender discrimination. They assure me that they only learnt of my involvement in the church after my transition became public knowledge and it was all just pure coincidence. Despite all those heavily publicised events held in my home after that police action and despite even at diocese level they chose to express opposition to the parish choice of me as their synod representative they still managed to remain ignorant of my involvement in church activities. Obviously I must respect their assurances it is not gender discrimination and that is it all just a coincidence. Quite what my wife has done wrong to earn such ostracism as well I do not know.

Fortunately my faith is with Jesus and not with a church establishment. My faith is with a God that in the scriptures tells us all that we were born with free will and free choice, not a doctrine that preaches "thou shalt do as I believe". My faith is with Christ who embraced sinners with love, not exiled and ostracised them from his midst.

As anyone who has had the misfortune to be a passenger with me in my car would know there is nothing gives me greater pleasure than cranking up the volume and singing along to the worship music that is inevitably playing, the misfortune not being having to listen to worship music but having to listen to me sing. My voice is lousy but it's the voice that God gave me so it's the voice I will honour him with!! I enjoy my relationship with God; it's a relationship of celebration, of fun, of deep love and compassion. I know of the love of God, I neither seek nor need approval from anyone else.

Chapter 15
From the outside looking in

This book largely centres on conclusions derived from many hours of psychiatric and psychological examination, counselling and psychotherapy that has helped me form my view of me and the events significant in my life or together the view of Jo and myself as we worked to overcome some of the many difficulties we have had to confront over the years. Sometimes it needs confirmation that the vision is clear. This is the view as seen from the perspective of three other people who were very close to us during the critical years.

Chris, who has been a close family friend for nearly 30 years and who helped Jo write her chapter, June, housekeeper and friend, who stood so close to Jo during the most turbulent period, and Nan, my secretary and friend, the person who telephoned me with the awful news that my home had been raided by the police and 2 ½ years later was dashing to London with Jo to try and find me, then an "at risk missing person". As with Jo's story each of these views are written either by the people involved themselves or by another person. In no way whatsoever have I interfered or influenced what has been written.

I wish I could. Reading these views have been an eye-opener. It's been repeated over and over again how I could be so overbearing, intense and serious no one would ever dare tell me what an arrogant rude pig I could be. Some of the comments that follow describe just that. I am humbled that the authors of these comments have been so supportive of me, so loving to Joan, I feel blessed beyond words over how they can forgive, embrace Jenni in their lives and feel ready to start all over again.

Christine's View

I first met David through my friend Jo. Our children attended the same primary school, so that makes our friendship 27 years old! Jo and I clicked from our very first meeting, and over the years we laughed our way through various jobs together.

We also socialised with our partners and children along with a couple of other families with boys of similar ages, We attended the Friday Night Drinking Club, the Sunday Lunchtime Drinking Club, and it seems there was always a BBQ at one or others houses. The boys got on well and it was such a magical time in our lives, like one big commune!

David was always the life and soul of the party, quick-witted and amusing, he was fun to be around. However, there was a dark side to David. For no apparent reason, he would fly into a rage over nothing, mostly directing his anger at Jo. No one could placate him, and he often stalked off, with an embarrassed Jo following him. David would never apologise or explain these outbursts, just acted as though nothing had happened, so we learned to ignore them. I often wondered why someone as successful as David could be so unpredictable.

Though they moved around the country, we always kept in touch, and we were thrilled when they decided to settle back in this area, where we could see them more frequently.

The BBQ's continued, but David was suffering from debilitating headaches, which would leave him writhing on the ground in excruciating agony. We felt so helpless at these times.

In spite of all this, David kept up his endless round of charity work, walks from one end of the country to the other to raise money for his various pet projects. He had endless amounts of energy and enthusiasm for whatever he was involved in at the time. Conversations with David were only about whatever project he was championing. From injustice anywhere in the world, the homeless, the handicapped, victims of domestic and sexual abuse, the list was endless, and no effort was spared in David's quest to put the world to right. Only now do I realise how little David talked about himself, or how he was feeling.

When that police action happened we were all devastated. We could not understand why the Police could not see that they had got it so terribly wrong. We all knew how strongly David felt about sexual abuse on children in particular. We knew that he had worked tirelessly to help these victims. I believe that in the past he had paid for the local Police to attend a course that was intended to help them to identify sexual abuse in children. My husband and I felt so outraged at this obvious persecution, that we, along with many others wrote character references on behalf of David, to no avail. For whatever reason, the Police fought hard to pursue the case, and a terrible injustice was done to an innocent man.

David has described better that I can how he felt. To his friends and family, it was obvious that he was severely traumatised. The impact this had on his marriage was clear to us all. He became impossibly overbearing towards Jo. I know she felt relief when he began to spend more time in London. We thought that it was only a matter of time before they would divorce, it seemed so inevitable, and there was nothing we could do to help them.

One July I received a letter from David. I hurriedly scanned through the pages and wrongly assumed that David was telling me he was suffering from a fatal disease. I quickly rang Jo, but could not get through. That's when I re-read the letter, and when I realised David was describing something called Gender Dysphoria, I felt huge relief! Is THAT all! Over the next couple of weeks, I often rang the house, and the strange thing was, I always knew if David answered in his suit, or Jenni in her frock!

We joked about how unfair I thought it that Jenni could have all the pleasure of being a woman without the the pain of puberty, menstruation, morning sickness, childbirth and the dreaded menopause! I wanted to meet Jenni.

I was terribly nervous of this first meeting. What if I burst out laughing? When I got to the house, it was David who opened the door, and I was faintly relieved. However, after plying me with wine, he disappeared without me noticing, and re-appeared some time later as Jenni, so I did not have time to feel any apprehension at all.

Jenni just burst in the room, poured us more wine, and started to cook our meal, it was that simple! Jenni looked fabulous, and the most noticeable thing to me was that she was so relaxed. I haven't seen David since, and do not miss him at all!

When I look at Jenni, I only see a happy, relaxed and confident woman, whose smile can light up a room. She manages (no doubt with Jo's help) to look better each time I see her! She occasionally gets the strops, but it is so easy to make her laugh, and restore her good humour. We enjoy "Girlie" evenings at local restaurants and Jenni relishes the camaraderie that only good friends can share.

Most marriages go through changes, from the first heady days of passion and lust, to balancing work commitments with childcare and keeping a roof over ones head. If you can remain friends through all the tough times, then the marriage can be said to be a success. Jo and David have succeeded beyond all expectation. Though Jo has effectively lost her husband, she has gained so much more.

Jo and Jenni have a much more equal relationship, based on real friendship and mutual respect. Both are happier than I have ever seen them before, and I just wish that Jenni was around years ago! I feel I have gained a good friend in Jenni, and feel so sad for all the years of pain she suffered being trapped in David's body, but at least she is free now to enjoy the life she should have had.

June's view.

June can be loosely described as Jo's housekeeper. She, like her sister Nanette, is also a cherished friend who has been a rock of strength to Joan during many difficult periods.

I have been Housekeeper to Jo and David for 11 years.

When I first met David, I found him to be arrogant and intimidating. I felt uncomfortable in his presence. If he entered a room I would feel it necessary to find work to do in another room.

I felt so sorry for Jo and wondered why she put up with him. Eventually, David's behaviour became increasingly more erratic; I shared Jo's belief that David was having an affair. I even suggested that Jo should hire a Private Detective and have him followed.

Things were very bad, the tension in the house was unbearable, and Jo was extremely depressed and unhappy.

Then one day, David handed me a letter, and left the room. This letter explained all about Gender Dysphoria, and suddenly everything began to make sense. I understood the pain David was suffering, and his unreasonable behaviour was a result of his terrible dilemma. For the first time a saw a more vulnerable side to David. I immediately went to him and said I would like to meet Jenni. David broke down. It was a deeply moving moment for us both.

I dreaded the moment, but about a week later I was introduced to Jenni for the first time. I immediately noticed that the hair/make-up/ clothes and posture were not quite right. But then we got talking, and noticed a totally different person. Jenni was relaxed, more confident and had a wicked sense of humour that was never apparent in David. I felt completely at ease in her company.

Over time her dress sense has improved tremendously, she now takes great pleasure in shopping for clothes, makeup and jewellery, and can't wait to show off her latest purchases. I would not want David back in this house, Jenni has become a real friend, and I feel totally relaxed and enjoy her company.

Nannette's View:

Nanette is my Secretary. She is also a friend, fashion adviser, provider of Kleenex and a friend again.

I first met my "Boss", "friend" and "Confidant" in 1998. I was then a struggling single mother who had just completed a business and administration diploma, with no foreseeable chance of employment in the public sector due to travel and childcare restrictions.

David of then was looking for a part time secretary and my name had been put forward by a family member. Trepidation followed, what would he be expecting from me, an ex psychiatric nurse with a tendency to want everything done yesterday, as nervous as one could possibly be and the knowledge that I tend to be a "bit" (poetic licence here) outspoken. David probably had visions of the head nurse from "One flew over the Cuckoo's nest".

Work was David's life, his charity commitments were endless and requests for his help and assistance especially in the area of child abuse flooded in on a regular basis. The work never stopped, this did take its toll at times and he endured regular bouts of cluster attacks. The obvious characteristic

Trapped

of David's personality always shone through even during the bad times and that was his ability to communicate. He had an ease and gentleness about him that was not always noticed by those around him. How many men do we know that could sit and talk for hours on what would seem trivial items, children playing up, husbands or partners giving us grief, down to having a bad hair day? David could and not seem awkward doing it. At functions, David always had the ability to be the strong macho guy with the gung ho attitude of getting things done and organised, but 9 out of 10 times, at the end of the evening he would be sat with the ladies talking home, family and women's issues.

I never had a problem or an issue with David, I enjoyed the fast go and get it attitude of business life, yes, we had disagreements and differences of opinions but we ironed them out in the office. David always noticed my sad days, always treated me as an equal and most of all we trusted each other and that's where boss, friend and confidant comes from.

The police action was a time of great sadness and disbelief. Nevertheless, it happened and I do not want to dwell on it as I could probably go on and on and it would achieve nothing. The knock on effect it had was heartbreaking to begin with, his will and wish was to fight but the compassion for others stopping him prevailed. This was then the catalyst to let his true self be born. David seemed to be coping but I new something was not right, he was spending more and more time away in the city and an intuition of him wanting to tell me something but never being able to do so was always lingering in the air.

This went on for months and months, consensus in the house was that David was having an affair, this did not sit well with me, as it just did not feel or ring true. The truth to David's behaviour was soon to unfold, by using the word truth, I am not suggesting he was lying; he was just not able to share his complex metamorphosis with those he loved dearly. Each time I came into the office and David was home their was a deep sense of sadness and loneliness, I thought being his friend he would open up but the time was not right and in hindsight I can see that the person most dear to him, his wife, had to be the one to tell first.

It was an ordinary day just like any other, which started the beginning of Jen's presence in our lives. I received a phone call from Jo, mid morning, she sounded very distressed and began telling me about a recorded message on David's phone, I said I would phone the mobile and hear what it had to say. The details are not important but it was a harrowing message of a sad suicidal man. Jo wanted to go to the city and find him, so I went with her. Her will power, love and deep concern got us to the city safely, albeit we smoked continuously all the way. Unable to find David we went to the police station, Jo let them listen to the message and they too expressed concern, so much so that they put out his details and car number plate over the police radio. David eventually picked up his phone messages and phoned Jo, he had to go to the police station and to cut a long story short, he was that bad that they suggested he section himself into a mental hospital. David and Jo talked for hours and in the morning, we all came home. Over the next couple of weeks, there was what I can only call a lull in the office and house. Something was going on but it was a secret.

Again, on an ordinary working morning, I came into the office and David had a brown envelope in his hand and asked me to read it straight away. "Good God" I thought I was getting the sack and he was handing me a letter terminating my employment.

I sat in the room and opened the envelope; I read less than the first page and said to myself "of course, why didn't I see it before". I read the rest of the pages, which laid out all what he was going through, the meaning of transsexual and

Trapped

why he had hidden these facts for so long. My first reaction was to give him a hug and say something stupid like "why didn't you bloody tell me sooner". David said something that hurt me at first "I will understand if you can not work here any more". Did he think that little of me, think or I was not a loyal friend; I ignored the remark and went up to the office. Sitting there and thinking on the past hour, I realised it was not David who had made the remark about working with him, it was Jen remarking on working with her, it was as if every bit of David's confidence had disappeared for that moment and I had been talking to a vulnerable, shy, frightened woman. It seemed so obvious now, all the little points I had noticed or seen but never put them together until now. Jen was home were she belonged.

Meeting Jen as Jen for the first time was a comedy of errors, Jo had invited us for dinner and Jen would be arriving later on in the evening. Sitting at the table, I kept telling my sister to call Jen, Jen or Jennifer. Jen arrives, walks into the kitchen and my sister says hello Jen, me and my big mouth blurts out "Hi David", Joan smiles, probably in shock and my sister goes red and I am oblivious to what I have said, unfortunately I said it at least twice more and felt the wrath of my sisters foot under the table. Did it seem unnatural? No, did Jen look fantastic? I will have to say no if being honest. Its like any learning curve, you get better at it over time and with experience. Jen has matured and grown, but we do not mention age, as like with any other woman it is our prerogative to be a bit vague with the truth when discussing age.

Because everything seems natural, normal or whatever word one chooses to use, I find it difficult to say what qualities Jen has, as the qualities David had are the same ones Jen has, what has changed? Jen has more laughter in her life than David did, she shops more, I can share a lipstick or a blusher and bitching about other people is now an office must. Ha Ha.

Jen is a woman, nothing more nothing less, her compassion and empathy is still there, her untidiness has not altered. Her love for Jo and family is unfaltering and has probably deepened over these past years. Do I miss anything? Yes. I miss the businessperson and the buzz of getting things done. This negative only counts in the office environment but I thought I should mention it. Jens priorities now lie in haute couture and enjoying life, I doubt if she really enjoyed life to the full before. I wish her and Jo health wealth and happiness in the future and I am proud to be able to say they are my friends

Chapter 16
Reflections

HEALTH: Migraine is a horrible thing. Almost certainly those headaches I comment on in chapter 2 were migraine headaches. I was diagnosed at 21 with suffering from migraine and all my adult life I have often entered a condition called status migrainous, where the migraine is continuous for days often requiring morphine to bring relief. The vicious neuralgia that brought my business career to such a crash and burn closure in 1988 was a weird out-of-control mutant of a migraine type illness called cluster headache and whilst it ceased to be chronic after about 5 years it still continued to be episodic, re-appearing for a few weeks before disappearing for months. I was unable to eat chocolate for all of my adult male years as it would trigger migraine. At the end of my male life I had a repeat prescription for specialist migraine tablets and injections and I was getting through prescriptions at the rate of 2 a month, 12 tablets and 4 injections.

When I was first diagnosed with cluster headache little was known about it. Now, today, it is known it is due to an abnormality in the part of the brain known as the hypothalamus. The hypothalamus is also the part of the brain that is responsible for sexual arousal and gender identity and it is the part that develops at 16 weeks of foetal growth and it is this part that develops abnormally resulting in Gender Dysphoria.

When I treated the Gender Dysphoria by going into transition it appears I treated all those other problems. At the beginning of this year I went to my doctor for another packet of migraine tablets. It had been 23 months since I last needed a prescription. Migraine has virtually disappeared from my life since transition and joy of joys I can feast off chocolate with complete freedom and abandon!!!

Other heath issues: Well, I no longer get regular attacks of mild eczema that required liberal use of cortisone cream on a regular basis. I eat far healthier, lots of fish, green salads, rice, pulses, bread with bits in it etc. I have lost a couple of stone in weight (size 18 down to size 14 and now possibly size 12) and I now get regular exercise walking miles, well, shopping for clothes can be hard work!!!

Alcohol: My dependence on alcohol as a crutch and to enable me to sleep really started around the end on 1996. Prior to then I always enjoyed drinking but I was able to leave booze alone when I needed to. Now, with the distractions to keep Gender Dysphoria repressed becoming less and less and my need to constantly search for other ways to fill the gaps of available time it became a crutch.

It did not help that our nice new house had a cellar and with my typically obsessional collector mania I had to cram that cellar with as many bottles of wine as it could possibly hold. However alcohol was to become a significant factor in my life and for 10 years there was hardly one day when alcohol did not pass between my lips, sometimes in a small measure, often in a large measure.

I would not call myself an alcoholic, very rarely did I drink during the day, sometimes on holiday, sometimes just enjoying a day out with Jo or friends, but never was there a need to drink during the day. Some days I did not drink at all. It was at night, when I could close the shutters on the day just gone, when I wanted to blot out yet another day of unhappiness, to forget, to find a crutch to carry me through the loneliness of night, a night when I would often be alone with just my thoughts, thoughts that subconsciously I had a great need to suppress. Often I would find activities to drive away those thoughts but those activities also on many occasions drove me to seek comfort from the bottle even further. They would involve perhaps a two hour long exchange of text between myself and someone, often in the USA, who had a need to express great pain and whilst they unburdened themselves to me I had no where to dissipate that burden other than through alcohol.

Jennifer emerging stopped all that. Now I have something to live for, now I can look forward to tomorrow. I have regular "LFTs", Liver Function Tests, as a precaution against any damaging effects that might be happening through hormone therapy and also to ensure that other past events that could impact on ongoing liver function are under control. so far they have all returned normal but I often wonder how long could I have continued along the path I was going?

First I tried monitoring the number of units consumed. When I was honest about it I was frightened to death to see how far into the range of "inevitable damage" I had sunk to. I started a process of reduction but still could not kick the habit of having a drink most nights and once that first drink had gone down the throat so the inhibitions and discipline often went out of the window.

Then, a few weeks ago, I was walking down Piccadilly just having left the hairdressers and on my way to indulge in much-needed retail therapy after a gruelling day of being pampered under the hair dryer. I was hit with that feeling I describe elsewhere, a feeling of overwhelming desire at being Jenni, at being me, at feeling normal, at feeling as free as a bird to fly now I was rid of that crushing weight of internal anguish. A voice inside me said "Jen, why are you killing yourself? Why, when every day now is so rich and beautiful, do you have to start it with a fuzzy head, lethargy and more often or not only get kick started with caffeine and pills? Jen, stop it, NOW".

So I did,. I am not suddenly teetotal, not become a born-again missionary of abstinence, but now I insist that for every day I take in alcohol I allow three alcohol free days to recover, that my average alcohol intake never extends beyond the recommended guidelines of 21 units and now my cellar is virtually empty, the source of temptation has been taken away. I have no idea what damage I have done to my liver, with TLC it will recover, all I do know is that now each day is not only beautiful, I can appreciate its beauty.

Looking back: I look back at episodes in my life now and think "Why in heavens name did I do that"? I then have to remind myself that person I was then; David was running, running from a deep fear of ever showing his real self. It seems all so daft now, so manic, so driven, so self-destructive. I feel sorry for David. Now I know the real him, the sensitivity, the compassion, the love for life and everything in it, but unlike him I can be relaxed, take life as it comes, be less intense and smile more. It is only now not having all that churning inside that I can see my life for what it was, never knowing contentment or peace. Whoever turned the lights out on David and turned the lights full on for Jennifer, thank you.

My life may have had its downs at times, it may have had its acutely painful moments but even the pain of the downs have been more than compensated by the fact all that churning agitation produced a fearsome driven energy that gained so much good for Jo and I. When I look at the downs and that pain I also realise that on the other side of the balance sheet has been a lot of good times, especially the good times of meeting Jo and becoming a Father to two great children.

When? The question I ask most of myself and others ask me most often is do I regret not transitioning earlier? Yes is the obvious answer but when? As a child, perhaps if I had been born 40 years later and childhood gender dysphoria diagnosed? Well, perhaps I could have had hormonal intervention, no beard to be painfully removed, no thickening of the larynx meaning no laborious speech therapy later, no testosterone build problems, but also No Jo, No children and what of my sexual orientation? How confused would I have been there?

So childhood may not have been the best time. When else? Another time Perhaps would be after that first physical breakdown in 1988? An attractive thought, we were financially secure, well established where we lived but could my sons have been so accepting then? They would be just 17 years old, a difficult time to have it revealed that your Dad is now going to be called Jennifer and is a she not a he. Could Jo of coped, aged 39? Could my body have coped? I was in dreadful pain, physically very fragile, I doubt it.

1997, when I had returned from my global wanderings and retired, again? Possibly this could of been the best time. In fact looking back this is when gender dysphoria had started to emerge from the subconscious where it had been so deeply buried. Had it occurred then, had that meltdown happened at this time I would not have been able to continue with my abuse survivors group, not become involved in providing support for abused and disadvantaged children and not been sucked into the spiral of events that led to being investigated by the police. However we were new to the area in which we lived and did not have the flat in London. Would this have made transition so much more difficult? Besides, in some ways that investigation was an accident but my involvement in helping so my disadvantaged and abused children was not and it contained many achievements I can feel proud about.

Personally as a Christian I have complete faith in Gods timing. It happened when it did, no point worrying, fretting or speculating on "what might have been" issues. Get on with it and enjoy it!!

When2: Now I have uttered all those brave words, and given one side of the arguments in my head, let me put a real emotion on paper. During one of my many examinations I was told "If you had only been born 40 years later you would have been easily diagnosed as a child". I just cry and cry every time I think of those words. Hormone therapy as a child, counselling to come to terms with myself as a child and not as a proud and well-formed macho male, delay of the onset of puberty until old enough, normally 18, to make my own decisions. No testosterone poisoning, no big, spade-like hands, no big feet, wide shoulders, deep voice, Neanderthal forehead, square jaw., no internal agonies for 18 months with thoughts of "blokes don't do this." I think of that peace and happiness I have in my life now, an ability to feel contentment that most people have and take for granted. I can only reflect on the years of pain and anguish I would of avoided. Yes, I admit it, when I allow myself to think of it the tears will not stop.

Ok, that's the weepy side to the argument, now pull yourself together Jennifer and be grateful for what you have.

Regrets: I am often asked what I miss most about not being a man. For me, personally, the answer is nothing. The only thing I miss is not being able to give Jo a man on her arm. The only regret I have about transitioning is what it has taken from Jo.

What I'm not often asked, for the answer is often assumed, is what I miss most not being born physically female. My answer is not the one expected which normally is that I would of avoided all those years of anguish and all those painful desperate months of transition. What I desperately, desperately miss is not being a Mum. This may sound strange, and don't expect me to have an easy explanation, for someone who was a Father and enjoyed being Dad to two growing boys but there is something that aches so deep inside me when I see a Mum with a young child, that very special bond of nurture, trust and protection. I ache so desperately at times the tears will not stop flowing but then, there are many biological women who have not been able to have children so stop being greedy Jennifer, you were a Dad, a very proud and happy Dad, so stop moaning and wanting your cake and eating it.

Still hurts though!!

Regrets 2: Looking back asking myself "what do I most miss about no longer being a bloke" and one thing really hits me hard. I actually have very little memories of being a bloke. As I mention elsewhere it is as though all my male adulthood had disappeared, as though I have resumed a continuum with that hurt and bewildered child of so many years ago, as if I have just resumed growing up where I left off when I left that child to prove to myself and everyone else I really was an adult male. My memories of being a bloke, what I did as a bloke, all the heroics and macho endeavours of being a bloke are fast disappearing from my conscious memory and in contrast long forgotten and repressed memories of childhood are returning.

Writing this book, recounting my adult years, recalling some of the most heroic, dangerous and physically demanding endeavours actually became hard labour. Not only did I have to constantly research back for hard dates and facts to act as points of recall, I was constantly bombarded with thoughts of "so what? What the hell is so significant? So you put your life on the line here, got a medal for doing that there, did bigger and better physical things than other blokes ever did, so what? Look who you hurt in the process, Jo, your kids, yourself, did you have quality of life? No. Forget it. Remember the compassion, remember the tears, remember the tender moments, and forget the rest, that's garbage. Remember that child, that child is now you growing up as Jenni Brown not as something that child hated and was frightened of.

Police: I am often asked about that investigation that blew the lid of suppression off the Gender Dysphoria. There is an expectation, especially from those who were close to events at the time, that I must harbour a great bitterness against the police. Do I? No is the answer. They were doing their job.

I am angry at the statements that were made to press and television, statements in direct contradiction of their own evidence, statements that could of put the safety of Jo, I and our home in jeopardy. I am angry that private and personal material could have become the subject of gossip in the small community where I live, surely a gross breach of public trust if nothing else and apparently condoned. However it is past, just another chapter in my life, something I have moved on from and something I will not allow to dent the happiness I have subsequently found.

The investigation itself seems to have been very flawed, just like the child abuse investigations in Middlesbrough, Orkney or Rochdale to name but three, it appears to have been an investigation that had got out of control and if it might have stopped the abuse of a few children it certainly destroyed the lives of a lot more plus their families. Over

40 people have died as a result of that investigation, taken their own lives rather than face the public hysteria and humiliation. I cannot speculate on what might have been found on their computers but it seems a hell of a price to pay if it has just been someone initially attracted to "Lolita" advertising and then developed a fascination.

The initial evidence that led to 6,600 homes being targeted for a "knock on the door" was flawed. In the United States the equivalent investigation that had 39,000 names on the list was halted after just over 300 arrests. It was halted because the original assertion that landslide was a child porn website was untrue. Landslide was a website that processed credit card transactions for a number of websites. It was merely a gateway, you paid the money to Landslide who in turn allowed access to those other websites. The vast majority of websites were perfectly legal therefore the majority of transactions were also innocent. Further, it was also discovered that significant hacking into the Landslide data base had taken place and fraud perpetrated, almost certainly what happened in my case.

In the UK the investigation went on regardless. 6,600 families were to have their lives tainted forever for even if later found innocent the damage had been done. Every statement made by the prosecution in court, every statement made by the media, every statement made by the home office all implied that Landslide was a child-porn website and the only reason people would subscribe to it was to access child porn, something which now turns out not to have been the case.

Perhaps one day the Home Office will let us know the results. Not just how many convictions, but convictions for what. How many people for example were found to either be physically harming children or had an active interest in harming children. How many took delight in seeing children being used sexually or being hurt in other ways and how many were convicted not of "landslide related" images but of accessing Lolita websites that were plying their trade openly and with the knowledge of a home office that did nothing to protect its citizens from accessing it? How many were convicted of having had material freely accessible on public domain rubbish bins?

Silver linings: There is another reflection I would like to make about that investigation. It is possible that it saved my life. Since 1997 my finger had been firmly on the self-destruct button. Every year there had to be something more, something bigger, and something more demanding to get my teeth into. How long could I of gone without pushing myself over the edge? I could not even drive down the M4 without exceeding 100 miles an hour, as a police video taken from an unmarked police car would later demonstrate in court! I was resorting to alcohol more and more to blot out whatever was driving me and we now know what that was. It couldn't have gone on much longer and the next breakdown may have well been my last. What is certain is that invasion into my home and privacy ultimately resulted in me being freed from my prison and for that alone I could almost be grateful.

That word: Well, I have managed to write the whole of this book without mentioning it. The word is **Transsexual** and it's a word I detest. However medically I am transsexual, my medical records attest to the fact I have been diagnosed and treated for Male to Female Transsexualism. Originally coined as an adjective by a publisher of pseudo-scientific journals in the mid 1940's to describe people who wanted to change their sex it was adopted by the medical profession as an adjective used then to describe "the most pervasive and severe form of gender dysphoria" in the days when gender dysphoria was considered to be a mental aberration of a sexually mature adult. Since then is has become an accepted medical diagnostic term.

It has also become a noun, I am A transsexual in the same way someone suffering from epilepsy is AN epileptic, someone who is diabetic is A diabetic. In the same era I was brought up in children and adults suffering with Down's syndrome were called Mongols, people with cerebral palsy were called spastics and to be gay was to be queer and to indulge in gay sex was an illegal activity. We no longer, thankfully, have Mongols, Spastics or queers going to prison for their activities so why have "transsexuals"?

Why do I object to the name so much? First is the inclusion of those words "sex" and "sexual". They imply a sexual motive or sexual orientation and nothing is further from the truth. It is a medical condition caused by an identity incongruence, nothing whatsoever to do with sexuality, sexual practice or sexual orientation. In fact one of the side effects of hormone therapy is to reduce sexual libido to nothing. That certainly applies to me, I have very little sexual arousal and hormones have rendered me infertile.

My second objection is that is sounds too much like Transvestite. I have nothing against transvestism and many transvestites have been very helpful to me but at the end of the day they are portrayed as people indulging in a recreation. Commonly used definitions of a Transvestite is "someone who from time to time adopts the persona and dress of the opposite sex for reasons of emotional release or sexual or fetishist pleasure but are otherwise happy to continue living in their assigned gender". It is a world apart from the pain and trauma of severe gender dysphoria, from the huge sacrifices so many Transsexual people have to make to just have a life and also just associates people such as myself with the world of drag queens and the exaggerated toilet humour of many area's of media.

I understand that many transvestites have a very deep need to give way to that female side, that they live with a degree of gender dysphoria and without that emotional release theirs would be an unhappy world but it is a release and not a need and I am not looking to give way to a strong female side, I am a female.

What else would I like to be called? How about Female, simply that? If it has to be qualified to explain I was not originally recognised and raised as a female, I was someone born with a birth deformity that prevented her from carrying out the biological sexual role of a female and instead had to behave as a male, how about Gender Dysphoric female, i.e. a person who was born with Gender Dysphoria but has resolved the inner conflict by living her life as her brain was made, not as her body was made? Perhaps this is too simple for a society that seems to want to place everything in tidy little boxes with tidy little labels on them but why does it need elaborating with an insulting misleading piece of ancillary terminology?

Transvestism: I make comments above that I wish to be distanced from the popular conception of transvestic behaviour but something I should make clear, so do many transvestites, not with the world of transvestism but from the popular salacious image that surrounds it.

In the classic but sterile description above, of people dressing for fetish, sexual or emotional release, I need to make it clear that whilst there are very many Transvestites who do just that there are also many who probably do not fit into such a sterile clinical description.

I know of many who's world would be one of deep despair if they cannot have that release, that there are many who agonise, just as I did, over the quandary they may be indulging in what is often portrayed as a sleazy or unnatural compulsion, there are those who find such genuine happiness in releasing their female side it must be asked "so why cannot society just accept that?". I have no idea why society cannot. Whilst nature seems to delight in producing endless variety some parts of the human race, especially that in the industrialised western world, seem only to be happy when they are confining people to tight narrow boxes of conformity.

In the past decade there has been massive strides in understanding the causes of gender dysphoria, especially where it affects certain people catastrophically, as with what is defined as transsexualism, but I think a lot more effort into understanding the needs of transvestites has to be undertaken and a lot more education of society needs to take place to be able fully to accept people for who they are, not how they present themselves. Everyone has a right to happiness and if it hurts no one else in the process what is wrong or unacceptable in people existing in more than one gender presentation in order for them to be happy, emotionally stable and released from unnatural and artificial constraints. Females have been dressing in the socially accepted clothes of the opposite sex for the last 70 years without censure, why can't blokes?

Finally: As I finally felt this book was complete, as the last of the thousands of "last versions" had been emailed to the proof readers, I found myself in a restaurant in London. I was there to organise the final details of a big birthday party, the party I mention in my dedication page. The owner greeted me with the sort of handshake and kiss on the cheek acknowledging my taken-for acceptance as a female. A couple of people in the bar insisted on buying me a drink or two and of course I had to buy them one back, would be rude not to. Monika the beautiful and sickeningly slender polish waitress greeted me with a "Hi Jenni" natural off her head smile, a couple passing, seeing me in the place, stopped and came in to join me, a normal night in the life of Jenni Brown.

Having had a little bit more to drink than planned I left finally at something over midnight, having popped my head round the door at 8pm for a quick "10 minute chat". Walking back to my flat down a quiet side street I suddenly felt as though my feet were lifted off the floor as that Giddy unbelievable feeling of being so at one with myself hit me. My lips involuntarily muttered the words "Miss Jennifer Brown, Female". The smile spread from ear to ear. I felt like I was floating, I was just so happy; I could have floated to the moon and back. It's years since I first saw an official document or credit card that conveyed those words.. "Miss Jennifer Brown, Female". It's still like an unbelievably priceless gift of joy. Will I ever get used to it? I hope not.

Goodnight everyone, thank you for so much love, acceptance and belief. Love you all. Jenni.

Acknowledgements.

My dedication at the start of this page pays tribute to 120 people who have played the most significant part in my life. However there are many others, often through the most innocuous actions, to whom Ms Jennifer Brown has much to be grateful for in terms of helping her become who she is. So, in chronological order of development, my thanks to the following:

Toni Louise. In chapter 9 I chronicle the most intense and desperate struggle as I fought to understand myself, what I was becoming and how I had to battle with all those conflicting emotions generated. One night was especially bad. In floods of tears, desperate to understand what was happening to me, I logged in to an internet chat room on a website for transgendered people and screamed for help. My cries were heard and answered by an angel. Toni that night held me through my darkness and pain. She convinced me I was not a freak, just Jenni, a female with feelings and emotions and a female who no longer wanted or could bear to go back into her prison. Toni, my heartfelt love and thanks goes out to you.

The Samaritans: Volunteers who volunteer not only their time but put their emotions on the line for the caller, no matter what the distress, what the cause of that distress is. Probably being a total over the top drama queen to say they saved my life but all I will say was that at the lowest point of my life they were there, they talked, they listened, they gave me a breathing space and a precious slice of time in which I could express my darkest fears, my darkest secrets, in complete safety and without judgement.

David Hawley, Counsellor and Psychotherapist: David was the person who I turned to, described at the end of my emergence chapter, to help me make sense of who I was and what I had to become. David confronted my two opposing personalities, broke them down and rebuilt them brick by brick, but rebuilt them as one person, a person who is proud of what he was and who she is. On my website I say think you to David for saving my sanity and possibly my life. I do not consider that to be an overstatement.

Warwick Whelan, Consultant, Torbay Gender Identity Clinic. It was Warwick that Jo turned to for help, who I met and was comforted and counselled by, it was Warwick that gave us both hope that we could navigate the dark tunnel we were in and come out into sunny daylight, together, our relationship still intact. It was Warwick who finally referred me to Doctor Reed bringing to an end a self-destructive period of semi denial..

Doctor Russell Reed. Doctor Reed was the one who not only ultimately diagnosed me as Gender Dysphoric, needing treatment for primary male to female transsexualism, Doctor Reed, in his no–nonsense kiwi style gave me dignity, reassured me I am not a freak, gave me hope, courage and guidance. Thank you Doctor Reed, as so many of your patients would testify, you are not only an outstanding doctor, you are an outstanding human being.

The staff at the Café Rouge, Chiswick High Road. In the days when I first ventured out on my own, it was to the café rouge I would often go, to sit in a corner, at the back, where it was dark, the least noticeable part of the restaurant. Despite at times looking what must to anyone of been a hideous caricature the staff always treated me with courtesy and friendliness, through them I gained confidence and a window of freedom in having somewhere to go.

Lorraine and all her colleagues at Marks and Spencer food outlet, M4. That first occasion that I drove home from London to Somerset as Jenni, described in the Transition Chapter, was a true milestone. My very early days of the Real life test, days full of anxiety and apprehension, just to be able to walk in to a strange place and be treated as just another customer, the warmth of the smile, the friendliness of the greeting, the courtesy extended to someone who was a customer same as everyone else. It all sounds so mundane and innocuous but for me was a liberating moment and something that will never be forgotten.

Mr V Deveraj, Exeter Nuffield hospital. I was terrified when I saw Mr Deveraj. I needed cosmetic surgery to my eyes. A terrifying thought for someone with a phobic dread of general anaesthetics and an even more phobic dread of scalpel-wielding people. Mr Deveraj could not of calmed me more or do a better job than what he did. To be rid of puffy eyes and disfiguring growths gave me so much confidence with the very best of care.

Doctor Ash Palmer and all the staff at Perfect Smile studio's, Hornchurch. When I first walked in, still very early into the real life test, I was not just a patient, I was a patient with disfiguring front teeth that needed all the concern, compassion and professional care possible to help me understand the treatment necessary and to help me overcome my phobia's. Thank you Doctor Ash and your wonderful staff. I cannot stop smiling now, and no longer am I ashamed and embarrassed by my teeth, you have helped me through my smile release the sunshine that is glowing within.

All the staff at the United Kingdom Passport office, Ecclestone Square, London. It is not often that one can use the words compassion, courtesy, professional and helpful together in describing a government department but that was what greeted me from that first time I picked up the phone to enquire about procedures to that moment I stood with tears streaming down my face looking at my bright shiny new passport with an "F" rather than an "M" in it. Thank you so much for helping me pass through a minefield of documentation and necessary bureaucracy with dignity. Your compassion, courtesy, professionalism and helpfulness will be remembered forever.

Andrew, Stefan, Jo, Charlie and all the staff at White cliffs., thank you for looking after my hair. You are not only the best hair replacement and augmentation service in the business you treat me, and no doubt every other customer, as royalty whenever I go in, even if I'm only going in for a moan and a groan!! Thank you. My hair transformed my life, at one stroke I was made to feel more feminine, confident and able to partake in any activity without worries that I and my hair may soon become distant friends. I can comb it, style it, colour it and above all swish it!!